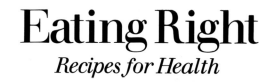

Eating Right
Recipes for Health

Fitness, Health & Nutrition was created by Rebus, Inc. and published by Time-Life Books.

REBUS, INC.

Publisher: RODNEY FRIEDMAN

Editor: CHARLES L. MEE JR.
Senior Editor: THOMAS DICKEY
Managing Editor: SUSAN BRONSON
Senior Writer: CARL LOWE
Associate Editor: WILLIAM DUNNETT
Contributing Editors: MARY CROWLEY, MARYA DALRYMPLE, MICHAEL GOLDMAN

Art Director: JUDITH HENRY
Designer: DEBORAH RAGASTO
Photographer: STEVEN MAYS
Photo Stylist: NOLA LOPEZ

Recipe Editor: BONNIE J. SLOTNICK
Test Kitchen Director: ANNE DISRUDE
Consulting Editor, Food: SALLY SCHNEIDER
Recipe Developers: SIDNEY BURSTEIN, AMANDA CUSHMAN, JACQUELINE DILLON, SANDRA R. GLUCK, SUSAN GRODNICK, MARSHA KIESEL, LORI LONGBOTHAM, WENDYE PARDUE, PAUL PICCIUTO
Food Stylist: KAREN HATT
Nutritional Analyst: HILL NUTRITION ASSOCIATES

Chief of Research: CARNEY MIMMS
Assistant Editor: JACQUELINE DILLON

Time-Life Books Inc. is a wholly owned subsidiary of
TIME INCORPORATED

Founder: HENRY R. LUCE 1898-1967

Editor-in-Chief: HENRY ANATOLE GRUNWALD
Chairman and Chief Executive Officer: J. RICHARD MUNRO
President and Chief Operating Officer: N.J. NICHOLAS JR.
Chairman of the Executive Committee: RALPH P. DAVIDSON
Corporate Editor: RAY CAVE
Executive Vice President, Books: KELSO F. SUTTON
Vice President, Books: GEORGE ARTANDI

TIME-LIFE BOOKS INC.

Editor: GEORGE CONSTABLE

Director of Design: LOUIS KLEIN
Director of Editorial Resources: PHYLLIS K. WISE
Acting Text Director: ELLEN PHILLIPS
Editorial Board: RUSSELL B. ADAMS JR., DALE M. BROWN, ROBERTA CONLAN, THOMAS H. FLAHERTY, LEE HASSIG, DONIA ANN STEELE, ROSALIND STUBENBERG, KIT VAN TULLEKEN, HENRY WOODHEAD
Director of Photography and Research: JOHN CONRAD WEISER

President: CHRISTOPHER T. LINEN
Chief Operating Officer: JOHN M. FAHEY JR.
Senior Vice Presidents: JAMES L. MERCER, LEOPOLDO TORALBALLA
Vice Presidents: STEPHEN L. BAIR, RALPH J. CUOMO, TERENCE J. FURLONG, NEAL GOFF, STEPHEN L. GOLDSTEIN, JUANITA T. JAMES, HALLETT JOHNSON III, ROBERT H. SMITH, PAUL R. STEWART
Director of Production Services: ROBERT J. PASSANTINO

Editorial Operations
Copy Chief: DIANE ULLIUS
Editorial Operations: CAROLINE A. BOUBIN (MANAGER)
Production: CELIA BEATTIE
Quality Control: JAMES J. COX (DIRECTOR)
Library: LOUISE D. FORSTALL

FITNESS, HEALTH & NUTRITION

Eating Right
Recipes for Health

Time-Life Books, Alexandria, Virginia

CONSULTANTS FOR THIS BOOK

Ann Grandjean, M.S., is Associate Director of the Swanson Center for Nutrition in Omaha, Neb. She is also Chief Nutrition Consultant to the U.S. Olympic Committee and an instructor in the Sports Medicine Program, Orthopedic Surgery Department, University of Nebraska Medical Center.

Myron Winick, M.D., is the R.R. Williams Professor of Nutrition, Professor of Pediatrics, Director of the Institute of Human Nutrition, and Director of the Center for Nutrition, Genetics and Human Development at Columbia University College of Physicians and Surgeons. He has served on the Food and Nutrition Board of the National Academy of Sciences and is the author of many books, including *Your Personalized Health Profile*.

For information about any Time-Life book please write:
Reader Information
Time-Life Books
541 North Fairbanks Court
Chicago, Illinois 60611

First printing.
Published simultaneously in Canada.
School and library distribution by Silver Burdett Company, Morristown, New Jersey.

TIME-LIFE is a trademark of Time Incorporated U.S.A.

Library of Congress Cataloging-in-Publication Data
Eating right.
(Fitness, health & nutrition)
Includes index.
1. Low-fat diet — Recipes. 2. Salt-free diet — Recipes. 3. High-carbohydrate diet—Recipes.
1. Series: Fitness, health, and nutrition.
RM237.7E38 1987 613.2 87-1970
ISBN-0-8094-6163-3
ISBN-0-8094-6164-1 (lib. bdg.)

CONTENTS

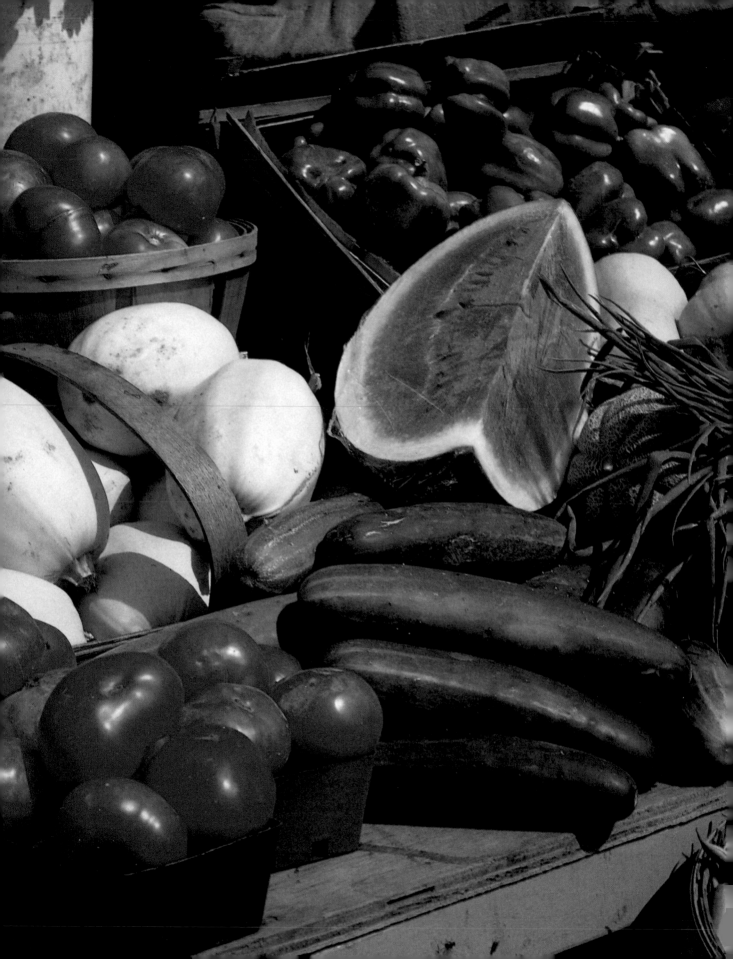

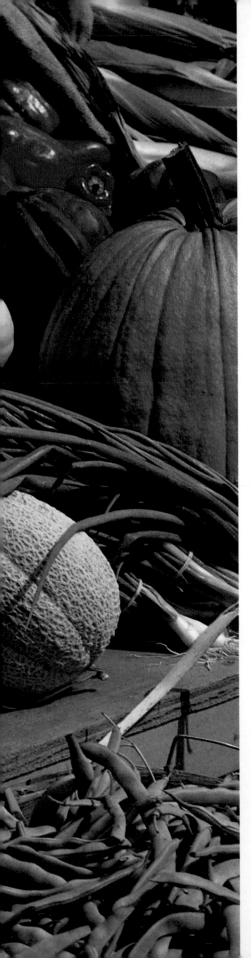

CHAPTER ONE

The Healthy Diet

*How and why the right foods — in
the right proportions — help you feel
more energetic, look better
and live longer*

To have the necessary energy and strength to get through each day and still have reserves left over, you must eat right. Some foods, because of their chemical composition, are more easily converted by the body into energy for your muscles than are others; still other foods contain nutrients that are especially important for the growth and maintenance of teeth and bones, and for the functions of the heart, lungs, eyes and other organs.

Food consists of carbohydrates, fats and protein, known collectively as the macronutrients, and much smaller quantities of vitamins and minerals, or the micronutrients. Water is a third type of nutrient in food. The macronutrients are used for energy and to maintain, repair and rebuild the different parts of your body. Most vitamins and some minerals help regulate chemical processes that take place inside your body; other minerals are involved in the formation of all your tissues, including your bones, teeth and blood. One of the most crucial functions of water is to provide fluid for your blood's circulation.

The Change in American Eating

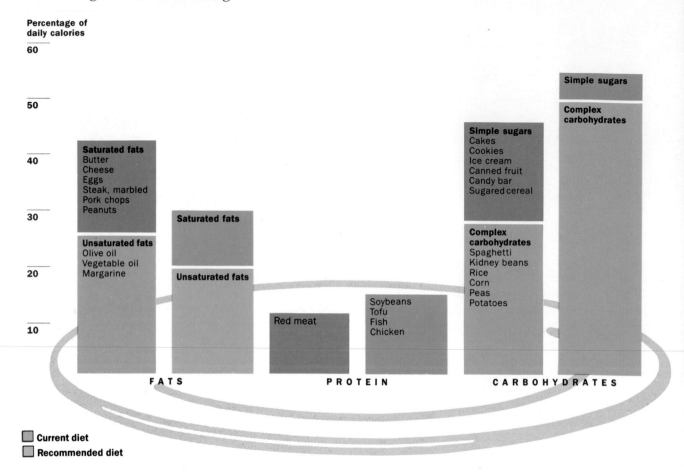

Percentage of daily calories

60

50

40

30

20

10

Saturated fats
Butter
Cheese
Eggs
Steak, marbled
Pork chops
Peanuts

Unsaturated fats
Olive oil
Vegetable oil
Margarine

Saturated fats

Unsaturated fats

Red meat

Soybeans
Tofu
Fish
Chicken

Simple sugars
Cakes
Cookies
Ice cream
Canned fruit
Candy bar
Sugared cereal

Complex carbohydrates
Spaghetti
Kidney beans
Rice
Corn
Peas
Potatoes

Simple sugars

Complex carbohydrates

F A T S   **P R O T E I N**   **C A R B O H Y D R A T E S**

◼ Current diet
◻ Recommended diet

Many people think it is hard to change their eating habits. But the American diet *has* changed. In the past few years, Americans have achieved the current diet shown above by reducing their intake of such foods as eggs, beef, hot dogs and butter. Taking this trend further will offer substantial health benefits, especially in lowering the risk of coronary heart disease. The recommended diet calls for reducing all fat intake by another 12 percent — to 30 percent of daily calories — and cutting back on saturated fat. The proportion of carbohydrates should rise to 55 percent and emphasize foods high in complex carbohydrates. Finally, protein sources such as fish and poultry should be substituted more often for red meat.

Developing healthy eating habits is not difficult; it merely requires choosing foods that offer the best balance of nutrients for your body's needs. In order to make the right choices, you need to remember these basic rules: Eat a wide variety of foods, get at least half of your calories from carbohydrates, eat high-fiber foods, consume a relatively small amount of fat and minimize your sodium intake.

Why are carbohydrates so important to eating right?

Carbohydrates, which are found in all plants and in most of the foods made from them, are your body's principal source of energy. Plants make carbohydrates from carbon dioxide and water; your body takes energy from carbohydrates by breaking them back down into these two substances and releasing the energy that holds them together. The amount of energy that can be taken from carbohydrates — or from fats and protein — is measured in calories. The caloric content of a food is determined by measuring the amount of heat produced when the food is burned in a laboratory device called a calorimeter.

The heat that is generated is analogous to the energy produced in the human body.

More specifically, your digestive system converts the carbohydrates in food into glucose, a form of sugar carried in the blood and transported to cells for energy. The glucose, in turn, is broken down into carbon dioxide and water. Any glucose not used by the cells is converted into glycogen — another form of carbohydrate that is stored in the muscles and liver. However, the body's glycogen capacity is limited to about three quarters of a pound; once this maximum has been reached, any excess glucose is quickly converted into fat.

Are carbohydrates the body's only source of energy?
No. Fat is also an important source of energy. Like a carbohydrate molecule, a molecule of fat is composed of carbon, oxygen and hydrogen atoms, though they are linked together in a different way. The body extracts energy from fat by oxidizing it — combining the hydrogen in fat with the oxygen that you breathe to form water, which releases the energy that held the hydrogen in the fat. This complex process not only depends on oxygen, but is also helped along with the by-products formed when carbohydrates release energy. As a result, it is very difficult for your muscles to use fat for energy without the presence of carbohydrates.

In addition, whereas producing energy from fat always requires oxygen, energy production from carbohydrates can continue briefly without oxygen. For that reason, only carbohydrates can provide the energy for short bouts of all-out exertion, when you are not breathing in enough oxygen to burn fat.

During a longer period of exercise that calls for endurance, carbohydrates supply about half the body's energy, while fat and, to a smaller degree, protein supply the other half. In fact, when exercise extends beyond 60 minutes, fat may provide 80 percent or more of your energy. But your body still requires carbohydrates to use the fat. Protein contributes very little energy; rather, it is the chief material used in building all of your body parts, including the muscles, skin, tendons, ligaments, blood cells and brain cells.

By weight, the energy value of carbohydrates and protein in food is the same — four calories per gram. Fat yields nine calories per gram. Burning a gram of fat, therefore, requires more than twice as much physical activity, and any excess calories that are not used in supplying energy are stored as body fat.

How are carbohydrates, fats and protein best distributed in a healthy diet?
If you divide the food you eat each day into its component macronutrients, the proportion of the total calories available from each should be roughly 55 percent from carbohydrates, 15 percent from protein and 30 percent from fat. These percentages are based on guidelines for a daily diet established by the American Heart Association, the

National Academy of Sciences and the National Institutes of Health.

To stay within these guidelines, it is obviously helpful if you are aware of the nutritional make-up of the dishes you are eating. Such information accompanies every recipe in this book. But reduced to its most basic elements, your diet will very likely be healthy if you avoid foods that are high in fat and refined sugar and eat mostly those that are high in complex carbohydrates.

What is so special about complex carbohydrates?

All carbohydrates are sugars, but they come in different sizes and nutritional packages. Refined or processed foods such as candy, cookies, jams and many soft drinks contain mostly the simple sugar called sucrose. These foods are dense in calories but offer little else in the way of nutrients. If consumed in more than modest quantities, they provide more calories than the body can burn up and the excess is converted into fat.

Complex carbohydrates are made up of chains of sugars that form the starches in a wide variety of plant foods, including such common foods as potatoes, pasta, bread, rice and corn, and a variety of vegetables and legumes. When digested, the sugar chains in complex carbohydrates are broken into simpler sugars. But unlike many foods that are loaded with sucrose, foods high in complex carbohydrates are usually rich in vitamins and minerals and may contain protein as well. Many of these foods also have appreciable amounts of water and indigestible fiber. Gram for gram, then, foods that are high in complex carbohydrates are almost invariably more nutritious and less fattening than sugar-laden foods. Fruits contain the simple sugar fructose, but they also contain the vitamins, minerals and fiber that many processed foods lack.

Don't you need a lot of protein for a healthy diet?

Although it is widely believed that large amounts of protein can make a person healthier and stronger, your body can take advantage of only a moderate amount of protein. Studies show that increasing protein intake above the recommended level does not enhance muscle size or strength; only the proper exercise can accomplish that. Even body builders on weight-lifting regimens will not benefit from extra protein.

Is meat the best source of protein?

All animal products, including dairy products, are considered complete protein sources because they contain all eight essential amino acids — basic chemical units of protein — that you need to be healthy. Vegetarian foods, which include vegetables, legumes and grains, usually contain incomplete protein, with one or more of the amino acids missing.

But it is possible to obtain complete protein from plant foods by combining them properly — generally, eating legumes along with grains or nuts. These foods, in partnership and in the right propor-

What is the best sweetener? Molasses can contribute significantly to your daily mineral intake by supplying some iron. Most other sweeteners, including honey, do not contain much of anything except empty calories. One advantage of cooking with honey, however, is that it is sweeter than refined sugar. In some recipes, you can add less honey than you would sugar and create desserts that contain fewer calories.

Time to exhaustion (minutes)

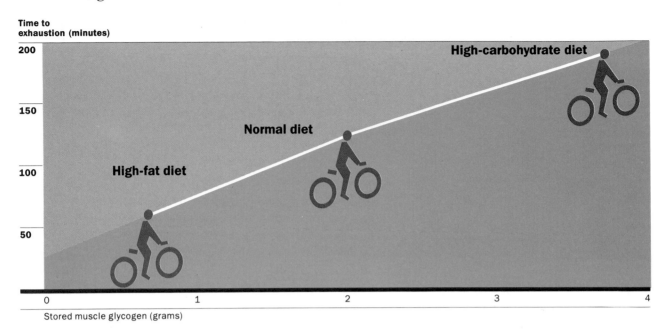

Stored muscle glycogen (grams)

tions, provide the complete set of amino acids sufficient for good health. Studies also show that vegetarian athletes perform as well as athletes who eat meat. And when you rely on plant foods for a good part of your protein, you can eliminate much of the fat that meat adds to your diet.

Should you avoid fat altogether?

No. Fat is necessary to maintain healthy skin and hair; it transports the crucial fat-soluble vitamins A, D, E and K; it helps you feel satisfied after a meal because it slows down the emptying of food from your stomach; and it supplies some essential fatty acids — the structural components of fat that your body needs, especially for manufacturing certain hormones.

What is the difference between saturated and unsaturated fats?

All fats combine two types of fatty acids, which are distinguished by their chemical structure and the relative amount of hydrogen they contain. Saturated fats are loaded with all the hydrogen they can hold, while unsaturated fats contain less than the maximum number of hydrogen atoms. Unsaturated fats, in turn, can be divided into two categories: monounsaturated fats and polyunsaturated fats. Polyunsaturated fats contain less hydrogen than monounsaturated.

Saturated fats comprise most of the fat in meat, poultry, shellfish and milk, and also include coconut oil and palm oil. They usually remain solid at room temperature and almost always harden when refrigerated. (The fat in most commercially available milk does not

A diet high in fat and low in carbohydrates not only is unhealthy, but it also lowers your energy. This graph shows the results of a study in which the same subjects ate a diet high in fat and protein, a normal mixed diet of their own choice, and a diet high in carbohydrates and low in fat. The subjects spent three days on each diet. As their carbohydrate intake increased, so did their level of muscle glycogen — the form carbohydrates take when stored in muscle tissue. With the rise in glycogen came substantially greater endurance: On the high-carbohydrate diet, subjects could ride an exercise bicycle three times longer than they could on the high-fat diet.

Cholesterol and Heart Disease

Initial heart attacks
per 1000 men
aged 30-59
over 10 years

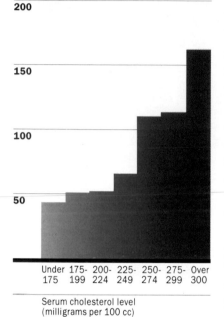

Serum cholesterol level
(milligrams per 100 cc)

Beyond a certain point, the higher the level of cholesterol in your bloodstream, the greater your chances of suffering a heart attack, as shown by this graph, which pools the results of several major studies. At levels below 180 milligrams per 100 cubic centimeters of blood, cholesterol is not a significant factor in heart disease. At levels above 180, cholesterol in the bloodstream begins to play a large part in the incidence of heart disease. Today, 80 percent of all middle-aged American men have cholesterol levels above 180.

solidify because it has been homogenized, a process that disperses the fat throughout the milk.) Polyunsaturated fats (including vegetable oils such as corn oil and safflower oil) and monounsaturated fats (such as olive oil and peanut oil) remain liquid at room temperature and when refrigerated.

Hydrogenated fats or oils are unsaturated fats that have been partially saturated with added hydrogen. The addition of hydrogen to margarine, which is made largely of unsaturated fats, causes it to solidify at room temperature.

What is the relationship between fat and cholesterol?

Cholesterol is a waxy white substance that humans and animals make from fat. Plants do not make cholesterol and therefore no cholesterol is present in vegetarian foods. All meat, poultry, shellfish, dairy products and egg yolks contain cholesterol.

In your body, cholesterol helps form the outer membrane of cells and provides an insulating sheath around nerve fibers. Although cholesterol is needed throughout the body, you do not have to eat foods containing cholesterol in order to be healthy. Your liver can easily produce all the cholesterol your body needs if you consume the recommended amount of fat (no more than 30 percent of your daily calories).

Besides its normal healthy functions, cholesterol can also form deposits on blood vessel walls — a condition known as arteriosclerosis, which, in its advanced stages, is the most common cause of heart disease. When these deposits build up so that they severely limit blood flow through an artery or cut off the flow entirely, the result can be a fatal heart attack or stroke.

Numerous studies have shown that diets high in saturated fat and cholesterol result in high levels of cholesterol in the bloodstream, while diets that contain a great deal of unsaturated fat tend to reduce blood cholesterol. Medical researchers have also identified cholesterol carriers in the blood that can more accurately reveal the condition of the cardiovascular system. Known as lipoproteins, these substances transport cholesterol through the bloodstream. There are two main types of lipoproteins: high-density lipoproteins, or HDL's, and low-density lipoproteins, or LDL's. By mechanisms that researchers do not entirely understand, LDL's deliver cholesterol to the body's cells, and in the process deposit some of it on the arterial walls; HDL's, however, appear to take cholesterol out of the bloodstream to the liver, where it can be broken down and eliminated. So although a person's overall cholesterol level is important as an indication of cardiovascular health, studies have established that a high level of LDL's is particularly associated with coronary heart disease.

Research indicates that diets high in unsaturated fat lower not only total blood cholesterol, compared to diets containing large amounts of saturated fat, but they also lower the level of harmful LDL's. (Diet appears to have little effect on HDL levels.) For instance, studies

Clearing Out the Cholesterol

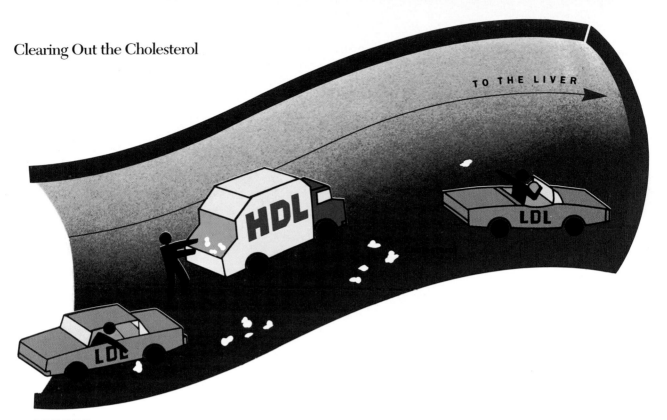

TO THE LIVER

ARTERY

LDL's (low-density lipoproteins) help carry cholesterol through arteries into cells; HDL's (high-density lipoproteins) carry cholesterol back to the liver to be broken down. A diet high in the saturated fats found in butter and animal fats causes LDL's to increase. As a result, cholesterol may be deposited on the walls of arteries, eventually blocking them and leading to cardiovascular disease. Lowering saturated fats reduces LDL's, thereby lowering the risk of a build-up of arterial cholesterol.

comparing Japanese and American diets show that the Japanese, who consume very little saturated fat, have much lower levels of total cholesterol and LDL's than Americans, whose diet is high in saturated fat. And Japanese who move to North America and switch to a typical high-fat American diet experience a rise in blood cholesterol.

What part does fiber play in a healthy diet?

Fiber is an indigestible carbohydrate found only in plants and foods made from them. It is not categorized as a nutrient since it is not absorbed by the body. But fiber adds bulk to the waste products passing through your digestive system, which helps to speed their elimination.

An excellent source of dietary fiber is the wheat bran in whole-grain breads and cereals. Bran contains cellulose, a form of dietary fiber that alleviates constipation and may help prevent colon cancer. However, you will be short-changing yourself if you use bran as your only source of fiber. Fruits, vegetables, nuts, barley, oats and brown rice contain other forms of fiber that appear to have other benefits, including lowering blood cholesterol level.

For a healthy intake of dietary fiber, most medical and nutrition authorities agree that you should eat a combination of foods that provide at least 25 to 35 grams of fiber daily — which is more than twice the average consumption in the United States. The following chapters will help make you aware of which foods are good sources of fiber. And eating the dishes in these chapters will ensure that your intake of fiber is adequate.

Mineral Friends and Foes

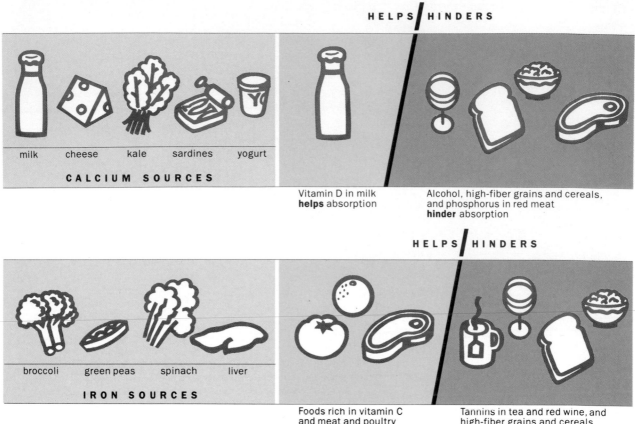

HELPS / HINDERS

milk cheese kale sardines yogurt

CALCIUM SOURCES

Vitamin D in milk **helps** absorption

Alcohol, high-fiber grains and cereals, and phosphorus in red meat **hinder** absorption

HELPS / HINDERS

broccoli green peas spinach liver

IRON SOURCES

Foods rich in vitamin C and meat and poultry **help** absorption

Tannins in tea and red wine, and high-fiber grains and cereals **hinder** absorption

The combination of foods that you eat during a meal can affect how well you absorb minerals. For instance, the vitamin D in fortified milk helps your body absorb calcium. But substances in alcohol, high-fiber foods and red meat all hinder calcium intake. Likewise, foods rich in vitamin C and animal foods enhance the absorption of iron from plant sources, while the tannins in tea and red wine and the fiber in grains decrease absorption.

Should you take vitamin and mineral supplements?

Many Americans apparently think so; between 35 and 40 percent of the population take a daily supplement. But if you are a healthy person who eats a well-balanced diet, you probably do not need any supplements at all. No study has ever conclusively proved that using supplements will let you live longer or perform better, lower your stress level, improve your sex life or cure a cold or any other illness. In a few special cases, supplements have proven to be helpful: For example, some women may benefit from taking supplements if they are pregnant or menstruate heavily.

Unfortunately, many people take supplements in the belief they will compensate for an inadequate diet. They will not. Vitamins only work with other nutrients contained in the food you eat. They cannot replace food or turn a bad diet into a good one.

Do athletes or people who exercise a great deal need a special diet to give them more energy?

Usually not. Studies show that consuming special foods or beverages or "loading up" on carbohydrates or protein does not improve strength, power or endurance. Because of their increased energy needs, athletes may need to eat more food than the average person. But the balanced diet recommended in this book supplies all the nutrients essential for fueling exercise and athletic performance.

Some researchers and trainers believe that a special diet designed to increase the amount of stored carbohydrates — glycogen — in an athlete's muscles and liver can help prolong endurance during workouts or events lasting longer than 90 minutes. But whether carbo-hydrate loading can improve performance remains controversial. And most researchers do not believe it can significantly benefit anyone except elite athletes, who train intensively.

Can you lose weight on the diet recommended in this book?
All nutrition experts agree that your weight is significantly affected by the balance between the energy you consume in your food and the energy you expend. If you consume more calories than you use up in exercise and internal functions, your body stores the excess as fat. (A very small amount is also stored as glycogen.)

While the information presented in this book is not intended to help you lose weight, it is designed to be the healthiest eating regimen available, based on the latest nutritional research. If you are over-weight, you can lose weight by following this book's dietary guidelines, providing you also exercise regularly and generally reduce the *amount* of food you eat.

Can this diet help you live longer?
There are many factors, including smoking, exercise and the amount of stress in your life, that determine longevity. But switching to the low level of dietary fat recommended here and reducing your intake of saturated fat have been shown to lower blood cholesterol levels. And it is well documented that lowering blood cholesterol reduces the risk of heart disease, the leading cause of death in the United States. A 10-year study concluded that, in men whose blood cholesterol is too high, every one percent reduction in blood cholesterol produced a two percent reduction in the risk of dying from heart disease. Another study of more than 350,000 middle-aged men found that the number of deaths from heart disease increased steadily as blood cholesterol levels rose, even when such other factors as age, smoking and hyper-tension were taken into account.

What is the best way to start eating right?
Scrutinize your daily diet. Begin by answering the self-assessment questions on the next two pages. After that, the information on pages 18-25 will help you gauge the value of what you have been eating for breakfast, lunch, dinner and snacks — and provide strategies for mak-ing your meals and snacks as nutritious as possible. From there, you can move on more knowledgeably to the recipes themselves.

S pecial high-nutrient sports drinks are promoted as helping to restore your energy. But according to a report from the American Dietetic Association, the primary nutrient that you need to replace when exercising is plain water. Rather than waiting until you are thirsty, drink a glass of water 20 minutes before you exercise, at 20-minute intervals during exercise and again after you exercise. And drink cool water — it is absorbed more efficiently than warm water.

How to Design Your Own Program

Even if you know that you ought to cut down on fat and cholesterol, watch your sodium intake and get enough fiber in your diet, you may not know how to apply these principles to your daily diet. It is easy to underestimate how much meat you are eating, or how often you have eggs or a dish of ice cream. To help you evaluate your eating habits — and become more conscious of them — try answering the questions in the box to the right.

Are you eating right?

1 **Do you use butter or margarine?**

Three out of four Americans now use margarine regularly because they think it is better for them than butter. Are they right? Margarine does have a nutritional advantage: Many margarines have at least twice as much polyunsaturated fat as saturated; the fat in butter is mostly saturated. And while a tablespoon of butter contains 32 milligrams of cholesterol, most margarines have none.

But if your overall diet is healthy, it actually does not make much difference whether you choose butter or margarine. The point is that if you keep the total amount of fat you consume relatively low, butter in small amounts — as in the recipes in this book — is no worse for you than margarine. Both have the same amount of calories and fat. People on a strict low-cholesterol diet are better off using margarine or a polyunsaturated vegetable oil such as corn, safflower or sesame oil. Otherwise, if you prefer the taste of butter, go ahead and use it. You can also try one of the new butter-margarine blends, which offer the taste of butter without as much saturated fat and cholesterol.

2 **Do you enjoy making your own lunch at a salad bar?**

Salad bars are usually stocked with a good variety of fresh fruits and vegetables, as well as grains and beans, which together can provide a far more nutritious lunch than a ham and cheese sandwich and a bag of potato chips. But many salad bars also offer such choices as seafood, chicken and pasta salads drenched in mayonnaise, which is 99 percent fat. And with only two dollops of commercial blue-cheese dressing on your Romaine, you may take in 16 grams of fat. You would do better to use vinegar and olive oil or, better yet, just sprinkle lemon juice on your lettuce.

3 **Do you drink enough water?**

On average, you will lose two to three quarts of fluid a day through perspiration, moisture exhaled through the lungs and bodily excretions. If you work out in hot weather, you can lose as much as two or three gallons of water in an afternoon. Drinking alcoholic beverages or coffee can lead to excess water loss, too. All this fluid must be replaced. You will replace some fluid by eating fruits and vegetables, which consist mostly of water, but you need to drink six to eight glasses of pure liquid as well. Some of this fluid can come from soups, juices and milk, but some should come from plain water.

4 **Do you drink some form of alcohol every day?**

In moderation, alcohol probably is not bad for you. In fact, recent studies have shown that people who drink two alcoholic beverages a day have a slightly lower risk of heart disease than those who are teetotalers. (Why this is so has not been conclusively demonstrated; alcohol may help clear cholesterol from your arteries and therefore decrease the risk of heart disease.) So, if you drink moderately, you may be doing yourself some good. But if you do drink, bear in mind that alcoholic beverages contain a surprisingly high number of calories. A can of beer, for example, has 150 calories — more than a small chocolate brownie; a glass of white wine has 80 calories; a vodka martini has 140 calories, plus another seven calories of fat if you add an olive.

If you are a teetotaler, no one suggests that you start drinking. There are better ways — diet, exercise and stress control, among them — to reduce your risk of heart disease.

5 How many times a week do you eat meat?

Millions of Americans eat meat for dinner almost every night, with a strong preference for beef. In addition, they eat meat in sizable portions — and therein lies the problem. If you eat half a pound of steak or hamburger, you are getting anywhere from 300 to 800 calories from fat alone, mainly saturated fat. And the amount of protein in an eight-ounce serving of meat is two or three times what you need at a single meal. A healthy diet does not require that you forgo eating meat. But you can get roughly half of the protein you need for a day in a three-ounce portion of lean meat. Substituting fish or chicken can cut down on saturated fat even further, as can getting more of your protein from plant foods such as dried beans, pasta, rice and corn. For guidelines on serving meat at dinner, see page 22.

6 Do you have dessert every day?

Pies, cakes and cookies are a leading source of the 100 to 125 pounds of sugar that the average American consumes each year. That adds up to 220,000 nutritionally poor calories — enough to make 62 pounds of body fat per person. You need not cut out all these calories. But instead of eating a slice of cake or pie that contains 200 to 500 calories, reach for a piece of fruit. Half a cantaloupe, for example, has 50 calories and a cup of strawberries has only 45 — along with a whole day's worth of vitamin C. Or you can end a meal with a yogurt-berry parfait (four ounces of plain lowfat yogurt has 72 calories). If you are an ice cream lover, try switching to water-based sherbet or sorbet — both have about half the fat.

Controlling your cholesterol

The fiber from apples, carrots, legumes, nuts, oatmeal and soybeans can decrease your serum cholesterol, while the fiber from wheat, bran, cereals and whole-grain breads does not affect your cholesterol level. Researchers also believe that the oil in fish may lower cholesterol levels. People who are concerned with keeping their cholesterol intake below the recommended level of 300 milligrams or less daily should limit their consumption of eggs — each yolk contains between 270 and 300 milligrams of cholesterol.

How to Read a Cereal Box Label

A product can be described as improved for up to six months after it has been changed.

The food's weight without the package.

Nutrition labels must appear on products that are enriched or that have health claims made about them by the manufacturer.

Nutritional content of each serving. To calculate the percentage of fat calories, multiply fat grams by 9 and divide by the total number of calories. For example, a dry serving of this cereal gets 8 percent of its calories from fat: 1 times 9 equals 9. Dividing 9 by 110 yields .082, or 8 percent.

USRDA percentages are general guidelines determined by the U.S. Food and Drug Administration.

Ingredients are listed in order of weight. This cereal has added salt, which you should try to avoid. This label also lists sugar and corn syrup separately, even though these both represent the empty calories of simple sugar. And, while these two ingredients are listed second and fourth, together they may represent the primary ingredient.

Crunchy Bran with Raisins

IMPROVED

ALL NATURAL

Net weight 12 oz.
(340 grams)

NUTRITIONAL INFORMATION

SERVING SIZE   1.5 OZ.
SERVINGS PER CONTAINER: 8

	Dry Cereal	With ½ cup Skim Milk Fortified with Vitamins A & D
CALORIES	110	150
PROTEIN, g	3	7
CARBOHYDRATE, g	29	35
FAT, g	1	1
SODIUM, mg	220	280
POTASSIUM, mg	200	400

PERCENTAGE OF U.S. RECOMMENDED DAILY ALLOWANCE (USRDA)

	Cereal	With Skim Milk
PROTEIN	4	15
VITAMIN A	25	30
VITAMIN C	*	*
VITAMIN B$_6$	25	30
VITAMIN B$_{12}$	20	30
RIBOFLAVIN	25	35
NIACIN	25	25
CALCIUM	3	20
IRON	50	50
VITAMIN D	10	25
FOLIC ACID	25	25
PHOSPHORUS	15	25
MAGNESIUM	10	15
ZINC	20	25
COPPER	10	10

*CONTAINS LESS THAN 2 PERCENT OF THE USRDA OF THIS NUTRIENT.

INGREDIENTS: WHEAT BRAN, SUGAR, RAISINS, CORN SYRUP, SALT, MALT.

MINERALS AND VITAMINS: IRON, ZINC, VITAMIN A, VITAMIN B$_{12}$, VITAMIN B$_3$(NIACINAMIDE), VITAMIN B$_6$ (PYRODOXINE HYDROCHLORIDE), VITAMIN B$_2$ (RIBOFLAVIN), VITAMIN B$_1$ (THIAMIN HYDROCHLORIDE), FOLIC ACID, VITAMIN D.

	Dry cereal	Cereal with skim milk
SUCROSE AND OTHER SUGARS, g	11	17
DIETARY FIBER, g	4	4
COMPLEX CARBOHYDRATES, g	15	15

Product name

Even though a food is labeled "natural," it can still contain preservatives, emulsifiers and unlimited amounts of sugar, fat and salt.

Whole milk adds another 30 calories, 4 grams of fat and 15 milligrams of cholesterol to each half-cup serving.

Breakfast cereals can add a lot of unnecessary salt to your diet. The 220 mg of sodium in this cereal is fairly high. You should try to eat cereals that supply less than 100 mg of sodium per serving.

Although the percentages of the daily allowance of vitamins and minerals in each serving may take up the largest portion of the label, equally important is the amount of fiber and added sodium and sugar in the cereal. Not all cereal boxes list these amounts, however.

Look for cereals with more than 2 grams of dietary fiber per ounce. This cereal, with 4 grams in a 1.5-ounce serving, has a substantial amount. However, the 11 grams of sucrose per serving is high. You should eat cereals that have 2 grams or less of added sugar per ounce.

Breakfast

One out of every four adults usually or always skips breakfast. Some researchers report that your mental and physical performance are likely to suffer if you do not eat breakfast, although other studies indicate that there is no effect on performance. But no matter how you function an hour or two after you have started your day, breakfast is one of the easiest meals to turn into the cornerstone of an excellent diet. All you need do is concentrate on foods that are low in fat and high in fiber, complex carbohydrates and calcium.

Unfortunately, some traditional breakfast foods are very high in fat and sugar, with bacon and sausages, donuts and croissants, and side dishes like home fries among the worst offenders. All the breakfast recipes in this book avoid excessive fat and sugar. But whatever dishes you choose, you can eat a more nutritious breakfast by following the steps listed below:

1. Omit the fat and sugar you add to traditional breakfast foods. Pancakes are fine as long as you do not smother them with butter, which is almost 100 percent fat, or maple syrup, which consists primarily of sugar. When you are in the mood for pancakes, try ricotta pancakes with strawberry sauce *(page 128)*: The pancakes contain a fair amount of calcium, and the strawberry sauce has vitamin C and fewer calories than maple syrup.

2. Instead of eating white toast with butter and jam, try whole-wheat bread with a lowfat topping of farmer cheese with fruit *(page 136)*.

3. To keep cholesterol at a healthy level, eat no more than three eggs per week. When making omelettes, add more whites than yolks; the yolks contain all the cholesterol in eggs. And cooking eggs in margarine or polyunsaturated vegetable oil rather than butter also reduces cholesterol.

4. When you buy ready-to-eat cereal, look for high-fiber brands that are low in added sugar and sodium. You can check the nutritional content on the cereal box, as shown on the opposite page. Combine your cereal with lowfat or skim milk and add sliced fruit instead of sugar for extra vitamins and minerals.

5. Cut back on the amount of bacon you eat and try adding more grains to your breakfast instead. The recipe for grits with dried apple and bacon *(page 48)* contains a good supply of complex carbohydrates and calcium and only a small portion of bacon. When you can, use Canadian bacon, which is lower in fat than other varieties.

6. You should eat a piece of citrus fruit or drink a glass of citrus fruit juice with your breakfast; both are high in vitamin C.

Remember, too, that there is no physiological reason to restrict your choices to traditional breakfast foods. For example, kasha-potato pancakes *(page 49)* and vegetable quesadillas *(page 128)* are just as satisfying to eat at breakfast as at any other time.

Lunch

At lunchtime, many people eat a cold-cut sandwich and a side dish like potato salad or coleslaw. But some of the most common sandwich meats, such as salami and bologna, are high in fat and salt and are often preserved with nitrates — chemicals that some researchers believe may be a factor in causing stomach cancer. A healthier sandwich filler is poultry, such as chicken or turkey breast, which is lower in fat than lunch meats. And a green salad is better than coleslaw or potato salad, both of which are often made with large amounts of high-fat mayonnaise.

With a green salad, choose a dressing that is not mayonnaise-based. The best dressings are made from lowfat yogurt, lemon or lime juice, or vinegar with a little oil.

Lowfat soups are not only nutritious, but have the added benefit of aiding weight loss because of their high water content. One weight-loss study showed that dieters who ate soup at least four times a week lost more weight than those who did not. Good choices are the white bean and corn soup, and the chickpea and escarole soup on page 80. While the beef, cabbage and beer soup on page 114 gets a quarter of its calories from protein, it uses a very lean cut of beef in order to minimize the fat content.

Experts recommend that you eat a moderate-sized lunch. If you start the day by eating a good breakfast, you will be less likely to overindulge at lunch. The following guidelines can help you decide what to include in your lunch:

1. Although lunch, like your other meals, should contain a healthy amount of complex carbohydrates and not too much fat, it should not lack protein. One university study showed that a lunch extremely high in carbohydrates and extremely low in protein made subjects feel groggy — possibly because high-carbohydrate meals stimulate the release of serotonin, a brain chemical that induces sleep. But including protein in the meal reduced or eliminated this effect. An example of a good, easy-to-make lunch dish that combines carbohydrates and protein in excellent proportions is the bean, cabbage and apple sandwich on page 83. The complementary proteins in the bread and beans contain all the essential amino acids — that is, they make complete protein — and the bread and apples supply adequate amounts of carbohydrates.

2. In order to minimize your intake of simple sugars at lunch, avoid heavily sweetened desserts. Instead, eat fruits. Many of them taste sweet, yet they consist largely of water and therefore contain far less sugar than most cakes, cookies or candies. Desserts like poached pears with strawberry sauce (page 72) contain some sugar, but they get much of their sweetness from the fruit. If you eat canned fruit, buy varieties that are packed in water or in their own juice; these have one half to one third fewer calories than fruit packed in heavy syrup.

3. Lowfat milk and milk products are good sources of protein and calcium, and they do not contain a lot of fat. A cup of lowfat or skim milk with lunch will boost your calcium and protein intake considerably, as will lowfat yogurt. However, commercially prepared yogurt with fruit preserves often contains a great deal of sugar. It is better to buy plain lowfat yogurt and add your own sliced fruit or whole berries. You will then get all the calcium and protein benefits of yogurt, along with the

EQUIVALENT SOURCES

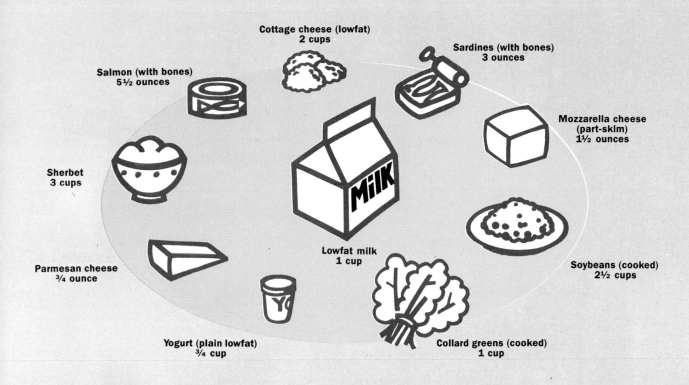

Cottage cheese (lowfat)
2 cups

Sardines (with bones)
3 ounces

Salmon (with bones)
5½ ounces

Mozzarella cheese
(part-skim)
1½ ounces

Sherbet
3 cups

Lowfat milk
1 cup

Soybeans (cooked)
2½ cups

Parmesan cheese
¾ ounce

Yogurt (plain lowfat)
¾ cup

Collard greens (cooked)
1 cup

vitamin and mineral benefits of fresh fruit — without the sugar calories.

4. The chart above shows foods other than milk products that will add calcium to your diet. For example, salmon and sardines, when consumed with their soft bones, contain a large amount of calcium. The salmon salad with lentils and rice on page 101 is a filling dish that is rich in calcium, has ample protein and a large amount of complex carbohydrates. Pasta primavera salad with salmon (page 107) gets most of its carbohydrates from the pasta, while the salmon supplies calcium and protein. In this dish, the complete protein in the salmon also helps your body take advantage of the incomplete protein in the pasta to boost your overall protein intake.

5. Avoid alcohol at lunch if you want to remain alert and be at your best for the rest of the day. It is a common misconception that a mixed drink or a glass of wine or beer at lunch can relax you and even make you more sociable. Actually, alcohol depresses the activity of your central nervous system, interferes with your mental capacity, slows your reflexes and can make you drowsy. It is also a concentrated source of calories.

6. Drink fruit juice or water rather than soft drinks. Plain water is the best way to replace lost body fluids. Fruit juices may have as many calories as soft drinks, but juices also contain vitamins and minerals. Soft drinks usually have only sugar, water and flavorings. Even soft drinks that contain fruit juice do not contain enough of it to counterbalance their high sugar content.

Drinking milk is not the only way to add calcium to your diet. The illustration above shows other food portions that contain the same amount of calcium as a cup of lowfat milk. The list below shows the amount of these equivalent portions that should be included in your daily diet.

Recommended number of cups of milk or equivalents to assure an adequate calcium intake

Children	3
Teenagers	4
Adults	3
Pregnant women	4

Dinner

Dinner is traditionally the main meal of the day, and the major part of that meal is often a sizable serving — half a pound or more — of meat, poultry or fish. If balanced with comparable servings of carbohydrate-rich foods, these protein-rich foods are not unhealthy. But when eaten too often or to the exclusion of vegetables and grains, large helpings of animal foods can cause a dietary imbalance by building up a surplus of both fat and protein.

Eating right at dinnertime can be especially problematic when dining out. As the sample menu opposite shows, many of the foods that restaurants commonly offer at dinner derive a great deal of their calories from fat. Whether you are eating out or at home, you can eat healthier dinners by keeping the following hints in mind:

1. Eat modest portions of meat, ideally between three and five ounces. You can do this — and still have a satisfying meal — by accompanying the meat with plenty of vegetables or by serving combination meat-and-vegetable dishes. The stir-fried beef with vegetables on page 113, for instance, has plenty of beef flavor but contains much less meat than a typical recipe for stir-fried beef or a serving of steak.

2. When possible, start your dinner with a generous helping of vegetarian soup or salad. In general, these dishes have fewer calories and much less fat than those that contain meat. By the time you get to your main course, your appetite will be somewhat sated and you will find it easier to fill up on less meat. A soup like the bean, apple and leek purée on page 82 not only gives you protein, but also contributes fiber, which meats do not supply. And when the soup is followed by a small serving of meat, the complete protein in the meat provides the essential amino acids that are missing in the incomplete vegetable protein in the soup.

3. Eat more poultry and fish than red meat. Without its skin, the white meat in chicken and turkey has less fat than red meat. And studies indicate that the fat in fish generally is not as harmful as the fat in red meat and may actually benefit your cardiovascular system.

4. Avoid using fat-laden cream sauces and butter to coat baked potatoes and vegetables — otherwise, you can turn lowfat dishes into high-fat dishes. Try combinations of yogurt, herbs, lemon or lime juice, garlic and onions.

5. Eat two or more meatless dinners each week. By combining legumes with grains — for example, in the lentil croquettes with spicy raita on pages 88-89 — you can get the same complete protein as in meat, but much less fat. Be sure, though, not to deep-fry these vegetarian foods or cook them with a great deal of oil.

6. When dining out, ask for your salad dressing to be served on the side and use only a modest amount. (Two or three teaspoons should be sufficient.) You can also ask for a lowfat dressing or mix your own oil and vinegar dressing.

7. Use the menu opposite to help you select main dishes in restaurants: The starred selections are all low in fat and include lean meats, poultry and seafood. Remove the skin from poultry and avoid foods that are fried.

8. Although fruit is an excellent dessert choice, foods like angel food cake and water-based sherbets are also usually low in fat.

DINING OUT
for Fitness

MENU WITH FAT CONTENT

When dining out, it is best to stick to dishes whose fat calories are about 30 percent or less of the total calories in a serving. The foods that are starred are suitable for a lowfat diet.

ENTREES	Percentage of Calories from Fat
POULTRY	
*Roast Turkey, light meat (skinless)	18
*Broiled Chicken Breast (skinless)	25
Roast Turkey, dark meat (skinless)	35
Fried Chicken, breast meat	36
Roast Turkey, light meat (with skin)	38
Roast Chicken Thighs	47
Turkey Pie	49
Chicken Nuggets	54
MEAT	
*Fresh Lean Ham	26
*Flank Steak	30
Lean Loin Lamb Chop	36
Cheeseburger	40
Lean T-Bone Steak	42
Lean Roast Tenderloin of Pork	46
Lean Sirloin Steak	48
Leg of Lamb	54
Salisbury Steak with Gravy	68
Pork Spareribs	80
SEAFOOD	
*Broiled Shrimp (no sauce)	8
*Broiled Cod, Flounder, Sole and Turbot (no sauce)	10
*Steamed Crab	18
*Broiled Lobster (no sauce)	19
Fried Fishcake	42
Deep-Fried Shrimp	43
Deviled Crab	47
Lobster Newburg	49
ETHNIC SPECIALTIES	
*Spaghetti with Tomato Sauce	8
*Bean Burrito	28
*Chow Mein	29
Beef Burrito	41
Pepperoni Pizza	44
Taco	48

SIDE DISHES	Percentage of Calories from Fat
*Beets	0
*Baked Potato	trace
*Green Beans	4
Mashed Potatoes	41
French Fries	48
Potato Salad with Mayonnaise	57
Coleslaw	87
Black Olives	97
SALAD DRESSINGS	
*Vinegar	0
*Lemon Juice	0
*Lowfat Yogurt	22
French	46
Thousand Island	85
Blue Cheese	86
Italian	92
Mayonnaise	99
DESSERTS	
*Gelatin	0
*Angel Food Cake	1
*Melon	6
*Strawberries, unsweetened	12
*Sherbet	13
*Chocolate Pudding	24
Ice Cream	49
Pecan Pie	49
Plain Donut	50
Cheesecake	57
BEVERAGES	
Cola, Root Beer, Orange Soda (but they do have one teaspoon of sugar per ounce)	0
*Black Coffee	0
*Fruit Juices	0
*Buttermilk	2
*Skim Milk	4
*Lowfat 1% Milk	23
Lowfat 2% Milk	35
Vanilla Milkshake	38

Snacks

Many people are led to believe that eating snacks is bad for them because the foods typically considered snacks — candy, cookies, potato chips and other so-called junk foods — are high in sugar, salt and fat, and low in quality nutrients. But snacks do not have to be nutritionally poor; nor do they have to ruin your appetite for meals or cause you to gain weight. In fact, if you are hungry between meals, it is usually better to snack lightly rather than not to snack and then eat too much at your next meal. The following suggestions show how between-meal snacks can supply important nutrients and actually keep you from overeating:

1. Avoid high-sodium snacks. As the chart on this page shows, snacks like potato chips, peanuts, pretzels and crackers, which are often liberally salted, can substantially increase your sodium intake. And too much sodium in the diet — more than 2,500 milligrams a day — can lead to high blood pressure, according to a number of studies. If you like these foods, at least find salt-free varieties.

2. Snack on foods that have not been highly refined and processed. Fresh fruits and vegetables, for example, contain more fiber and water than processed varieties, so they fill you up on fewer calories. Fresh foods also typically contain more vitamins and minerals and less fat. For instance, plain baked potatoes contain only a fraction of the fat that potato chips and french fries absorb during processing.

3. Choose crackers and cookies made with unsaturated oil. Many crackers contain palm or coconut oil, both of which consist of mostly saturated fats that can contribute to

Most of the sodium that you eat is already in your food by the time it reaches your plate and before you use a salt shaker. By choosing foods lower in sodium, you can decrease your sodium intake; the chart below shows examples of high- and low-sodium foods. In addition to eating the right foods, you can also cut your sodium consumption by using herbs and spices, instead of salt, to season your food.

Where Your Sodium Comes From

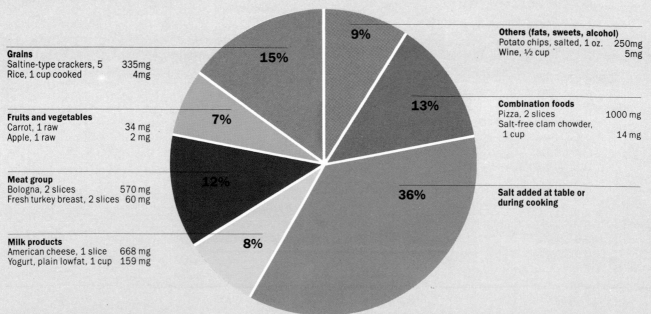

Grains
Saltine-type crackers, 5   335mg
Rice, 1 cup cooked   4mg

Fruits and vegetables
Carrot, 1 raw   34 mg
Apple, 1 raw   2 mg

Meat group
Bologna, 2 slices   570 mg
Fresh turkey breast, 2 slices   60 mg

Milk products
American cheese, 1 slice   668 mg
Yogurt, plain lowfat, 1 cup   159 mg

Others (fats, sweets, alcohol)
Potato chips, salted, 1 oz.   250mg
Wine, ½ cup   5mg

Combination foods
Pizza, 2 slices   1000 mg
Salt-free clam chowder,
1 cup   14 mg

Salt added at table or during cooking

9%
15%
7%
13%
12%
8%
36%

The Basic Guidelines for Eating Right

For a moderately active adult, the National Institutes of Health recommends a diet that is low in fat, high in carbohydrates and moderate in protein. The institutes' guidelines suggest that no more than 30 percent of your calories come from fat, that 55 to 60 percent come from carbohydrates and that no more than 15 percent come from protein. A gram of fat equals nine calories, while a gram of protein or carbohydrate equals four calories; therefore, if you eat 2,100 calories a day, you should consume approximately 60 grams of fat, 315 grams of carbohydrate and no more than 75 grams of protein daily. If you follow a lowfat/high-carbohydrate diet, your chance of developing heart disease, cancer and other life-threatening diseases may be considerably reduced.

The nutrition charts that accompany each of the lowfat/high-carbohydrate recipes in this book include the number of calories per serving, the number of grams of fat, carbohydrate and protein in a serving, and the percentage of calories derived from each of these nutrients. In addition, the charts provide the amount of calcium, iron and sodium per serving.

Calcium deficiency may be associated with periodontal disease — which attacks the mouth's bones and tissues, including the gums — in both men and women, and with osteoporosis, or bone shrinking and weakening, in the elderly. The deficiency may also contribute to high blood pressure. The recommended daily allowance for calcium is 800 milligrams a day for men and women. Pregnant and lactating women are advised to consume 1,200 milligrams daily; a National Institutes of Health consensus panel recommends that postmenopausal women consume between 1,200 and 1,500 milligrams of calcium daily.

Although one way you can reduce your fat intake is to cut your consumption of red meat, you should make sure that you get your necessary iron from other sources. The Food and Nutrition Board of the National Academy of Sciences suggests a minimum of 10 milligrams of iron per day for men and 18 milligrams for women between the ages of 11 and 50.

High sodium intake is associated with high blood pressure. Most adults should restrict sodium intake to between 2,000 and 2,500 milligrams a day, according to the National Academy of Sciences. One way to keep sodium consumption in check is not to add table salt to food.

arteriosclerosis. Healthier crackers — sesame sticks, stoned-wheat crackers, rice cakes and bran wafers — are made with unsaturated oils such as soybean, safflower or corn oil.

4. Make your own popcorn in a hot-air popper but skip the butter. If you use butter or oil, the popcorn absorbs most of it, more than doubling the calories and boosting the fat content substantially. To add flavor, sprinkle the hot popcorn with herbs, spices or a small amount of grated sharp cheese.

5. Unsweetened or low-sugar cereal eaten with lowfat milk or yogurt makes a healthy, filling snack. The recipe for muesli on page 65 is an example. Avoid commercially made granola and granola bars, which generally contain saturated fat in the form of coconut oil.

6. Soft drinks, which many people drink with snacks, usually contain flavoring, sugar and water, but little else. More nutritious beverages are made from fruit mixtures, such as homemade cranberry-spice, blueberry-vanilla or raspberry syrup (*pages 74-75*). These and other drinks made from fresh fruits contain vitamins, minerals and fiber.

Guide to Vitamins and Minerals

Vitamin	Adult RDA or Estimated Intake	Food Sources	What It Does
A	800-1,000 mcg (micrograms)	Liver, eggs, fortified milk, carrots, tomatoes, apricots, cantaloupe, fish	Promotes good vision; helps form and maintain healthy skin and mucous membranes; may protect against some cancers
C	50-60 mg (milligrams)	Citrus fruits, strawberries, tomatoes	Promotes healthy capillaries, gums and teeth; aids iron absorption; may block production of nitrosamines; maintains normal connective tissue; aids in healing wounds
D	5-10 mcg (200-400 International Units)	Fortified milk, fish; also produced by the body in response to sunlight	Promotes strong bones and teeth; necessary for absorption of calcium
E	8-10 mg	Nuts, vegetable oils, whole grains, olives, asparagus, spinach	Protects tissue against oxidation; important in formation of red blood cells; helps the body use vitamin K
K	70-140 mcg°	Body produces about half of its daily needs; cauliflower, broccoli, cabbage, spinach, cereals, soybeans, beef liver	Aids in clotting of blood
B-1 (Thiamin)	1-1.5 mg	Whole grains, dried beans, lean meats (especially pork), fish	Helps release energy from carbohydrates; necessary for healthy brain and nerve cells and for functioning of heart
B-2 (Riboflavin)	1.2-1.7 mg	Nuts, dairy products, liver	Aids in release of energy from foods; interacts with other B vitamins
B-3 (Niacin)	13-19 mg	Nuts, dairy products, liver	Aids in release of energy from foods; involved in synthesis of DNA; maintains normal functioning of skin, nerves and digestive system
B-5 (Pantothenic acid)	4-7 mg°	Whole grains, dried beans, eggs, nuts	Aids in release of energy from foods; essential for synthesis of numerous body materials
B-6 (Pyridoxine)	1.8-2.2 mg	Whole grains, dried beans, eggs, nuts	Important in chemical reactions of proteins and amino acids; involved in normal functioning of brain and formation of red blood cells
B-12	3 mcg	Liver, beef, eggs, milk, shellfish	Necessary for development of red blood cells; maintains normal functioning of nervous system
Folacin	400 mcg	Liver, wheat bran, leafy green vegetables, beans, grains	Important in the synthesis of DNA; acts together with B-12 in the production of hemoglobin
Biotin	100-200 mcg°	Yeast, eggs, liver, milk	Important in formation of fatty acids; helps metabolize amino acids and carbohydrates

The RDA, or Recommended Dietary Allowance, refers to the amount of a given nutrient required daily to maintain good nutrition. Each RDA takes into account individual variations among most normal healthy people with the exception of pregnant or lactating women, who may need additional vitamins and minerals. An asterisk (°) denotes that no RDA has been established for a particular nutrient, and that an estimated safe intake has been given.

Major Mineral	Adult RDA or Estimated Intake	Food Sources	What It Does
Calcium	800 mg (1,200-1,500 mg for older women) 1 quart milk = 1,250 mg	Milk and milk products, sardines and salmon eaten with bones, dark green leafy vegetables, shellfish, hard water	Builds bones and teeth, and maintains bone density and strength; helps prevent osteoporosis in older population; plays a role in regulating heartbeat, blood clotting, muscle contraction
Chloride	1,900-5,000 mg°	Table salt, fish, pickled and smoked foods	Maintains normal fluid shifts; balances pH of blood; forms hydrochloric acid in stomach
Magnesium	300 mg (women) 350 mg (men) 1 cup spinach = 160 mg	Wheat bran, whole grains, raw leafy green vegetables, nuts, soybeans, bananas, apricots, hard water, spices	Aids in bone growth; aids functioning of nerves and muscles, including regulation of normal heart rhythm
Phosphorus	800 mg 1 cup milk = 993 mg; 1 serving chicken = 231 mg	Meats, poultry, fish, cheese, egg yolks, dried peas and beans, milk and milk products, soft drinks	Aids bone growth and strengthening of teeth; important in energy metabolism
Potassium	1,500-6,000 mg° 1 cup raisins = 524 mg; 1 banana = 400 mg; 1 small potato = 400 mg	Oranges, bananas, raisins, peanut butter, dried peas and beans, potatoes, coffee, tea, cocoa, yogurt, molasses, meat	Promotes regular heartbeat; active in muscle contraction; regulates transfer of nutrients to cells; controls water balance in body tissues and cells
Sodium	2,300-3,300 mg° 1 frozen pot pie = 1,600 mg	All from salt	Helps regulate water balance in body; plays a role in maintaining blood pressure

Trace Mineral	Adult RDA or Estimated Intake	Food Sources	What It Does
Chromium	.05-.20 mg°	Meat, cheese, whole grains, dried peas and beans, brewer's yeast	Important for glucose metabolism; may be a cofactor for insulin
Copper	2-3 mg°	Shellfish (especially oysters), nuts, beef and pork liver, chocolate, kidneys, dried beans, raisins, margarine	Formation of red blood cells; cofactor in absorbing iron into blood cells; assists in production of several enzymes involved in respiration; interacts with zinc
Fluorine (fluoride)	1.5-4.0 mg°	Fluoridated water, foods grown with or cooked in fluoridated water, fish, tea, gelatin	Contributes to solid bone and tooth formation; may help prevent osteoporosis in older people
Iodine	.15 mg	Primarily from iodized salt; also seafood, seaweed products, vegetables grown in iodine-rich areas, vegetable oil	Necessary for normal function of thyroid gland; essential for normal cell function; keeps skin, hair and nails healthy; prevents goiter
Iron	10 mg (male) 18 mg (female during childbearing years) 4 oz calf's liver = 12 mg	Liver (especially pork), kidneys, red meats, egg yolks, peas, beans, nuts, dried fruits, leafy green vegetables, enriched grain products, blackstrap molasses	Essential to formation of hemoglobin, the oxygen-carrying factor in the blood; part of several enzymes and proteins in the body
Manganese	2.5-5.0 mg° ½ cup peanut butter = 2 mg	Nuts, whole grains, vegetables, fruits, instant coffee, tea, cocoa powder, beets, egg yolks	Required for normal bone growth and development, normal reproduction and cell function
Molybdenum	.15-.50 mg°	Peas, beans, cereal grains, organ meats, dark green vegetables	Important for normal cell function
Selenium	.05-.20 mg° 4 oz fish = .04 mg	Fish, shellfish, red meat, egg yolks, chicken, garlic	Complements vitamin E to fight cell damage by oxygen
Zinc	15 mg° 5 oysters = 160 mg 2 slices whole-wheat bread = 2 mg	Oysters, crab meat, beef, liver, eggs, poultry, brewer's yeast, whole-wheat bread	Maintains normal taste and smell acuity, growth and sexual development; important for fetal growth and wound healing

Major minerals are present in a healthy body in quantities exceeding five grams each. Trace minerals, or microminerals, are present in much smaller quantities, though they are no less essential to good nutrition. The function of some trace minerals is not understood; this chart lists only those trace minerals for which functions have been identified.

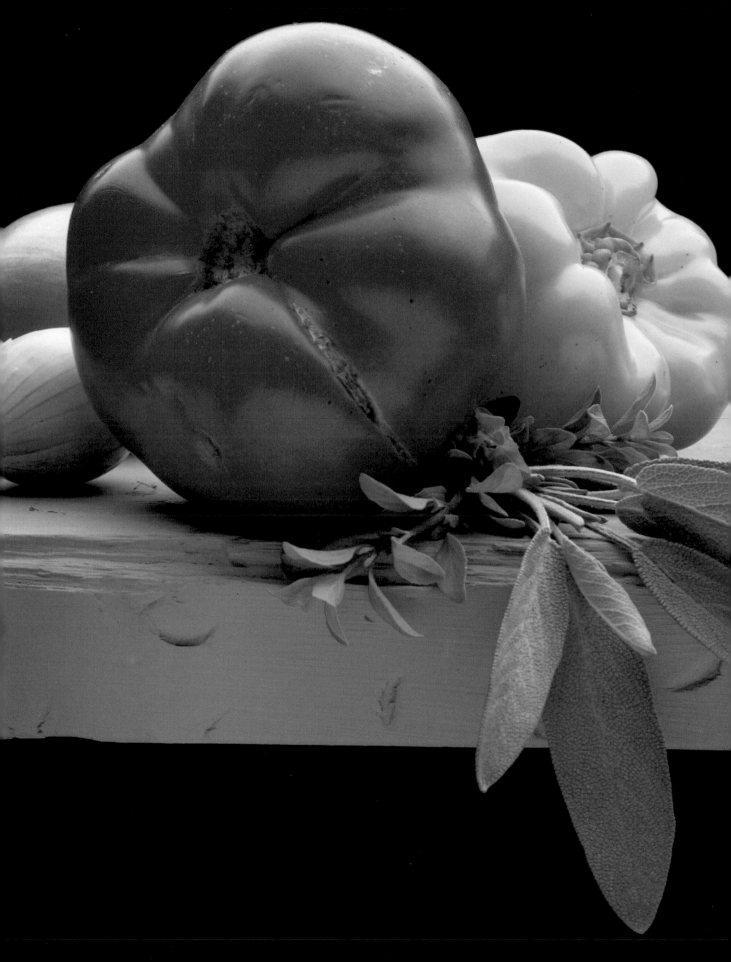

CHAPTER TWO

Vegetables

*Flavorful, colorful, low in calories —
and with abundant vitamins
and minerals*

Virtually all vegetables are nutritionally dense. For example, one and a half cups of Romaine lettuce can supply half your daily requirement of vitamin A in the form of beta carotene (which the body converts to vitamin A), a third of your vitamin C and almost 10 percent of your iron — all in only 12 calories. Three and a half ounces of collard greens — 40 calories — provide more vitamin A and C than you need daily, more than 20 percent of your daily requirements of potassium, calcium and riboflavin (a B vitamin necessary for energy production in cells), and about 10 percent of your thiamin and niacin requirements. Even half a cup of the starchiest vegetables, such as potatoes, squash and corn, contains fewer calories than a tablespoon of butter. Furthermore, most vegetables are low in sodium and fat and high in fiber, the indigestible portion of a plant.

Vegetables keep you healthy in several ways. A recent study at Johns Hopkins University showed that a high blood level of beta carotene, which virtually all leafy green and yellow vegetables contain, appears to reduce the risk of some kinds of cancer by protecting cells and tissues from harmful chemicals called free radicals. A diet with one or more daily servings of cruciferous vegetables, which include broccoli, Brussels sprouts and cauliflower, helps protect against cancer. Studies also show that certain vegetable fibers — lignins, pectins and gums — appear to lower serum cholesterol, may reduce the risk of arteriosclerosis, promote regularity and may guard against certain forms of cancer.

A vegetable's nutrient content depends largely on the part of the plant it comes from. The leafy parts of plants generally contain a great deal of water and very few carbohydrates; yet they supply substantial amounts of beta carotene, vitamin C and riboflavin. Dark green leaves, such as those of spinach and mustard greens, contain more beta carotene than do pale leaves, like those of iceberg lettuce. A dark-green color usually signals high calcium content, but because some dark-green vegetables contain oxalic acid — a calcium inhibitor — you should not rely on them as your primary calcium source.

Fruit vegetables, such as tomatoes, cucumbers and bell peppers, are the pulpy, seed-bearing part of the plant. They are slightly higher in calories than leafy vegetables and contain large quantities of vitamin C. Because their peels contain fiber and protect the vitamins under the surface, it is best not to peel these vegetables — or any vegetables with skins — before you eat them. If a recipe calls for peeling, peel vegetables as thinly as possible and just before you cook them.

Vegetables from the buds, stalks and flowers of plants, such as asparagus, broccoli and cauliflower, are low in calories and high in vitamins and minerals. Broccoli, for example, is particularly high in vitamin C and calcium; its leaves have four times the calcium and twice the beta carotene and riboflavin of its florets.

Root, bulb and tuber vegetables, such as potatoes, beets and carrots, have less water, more carbohydrates and more calories per serving than most other vegetables. Potatoes, both white and sweet, contain substantial amounts of vitamin C. The skins are high in fiber. And sweet potatoes and carrots also have exceptionally high amounts of beta carotene. (The average sweet potato supplies about five times the required daily amount of vitamin A.) The darker its yellow color, the more beta carotene a vegetable contains.

Before you cook fresh vegetables, wash them under a steady stream of water to get rid of dirt, insects, surface pesticides and bacteria. Sandy greens, such as spinach and arugula, should be soaked briefly in the sink, using several changes of water (long soaking may remove nutrients). Do not cut fresh vegetables until you are ready to cook them: Exposure to air destroys their vitamin C and A, while light lowers their riboflavin and vitamin K content.

Steaming vegetables until they are just crisp-tender makes them taste better and preserves more vitamins and minerals than boiling. Use a vegetable steamer or other container with a tight-fitting lid. If

Buying and Storing Guide

> In general, yellow and green vegetables that are dark, young and small have the best taste and the most nutrients. Fresh vegetables are usually the best nutritional buy and frozen are second best. Canned vegetables — which lose taste, consistency and nutrients during high-heat processing — should be your last choice. For the best quality and value, buy vegetables in season and shop at roadside farm stands whenever possible.

> When shopping in supermarkets, buy unwrapped produce that you can inspect and select individually. Prewrapped items may be damaged or of inconsistent quality. Check to see that no part of a vegetable is damaged or wilted. Aging and bruising release enzymes that lower the vitamin content.

> Buy no more than you will eat in a few days: As soon as vegetables have been picked, their natural sugar begins to change to starch and they begin to lose their sweetness. Most vegetables should be stored in the refrigerator until you are ready to eat them. After buying root vegetables, such as beets or carrots, remove their tops right away; otherwise, their leaves will let moisture escape. Tomatoes should be allowed to ripen at room temperature before they are refrigerated. White potatoes, sweet potatoes and onions should be kept in a well-ventilated place that is cool, dark and dry.

> You can freeze many fresh vegetables and preserve most of their nutrients. But if you freeze vegetables after cooking them, they will be soft, less tasty and less nutritious when you reheat them. Cooked vegetables can be kept refrigerated for about five days: Store them in plastic bags or tightly covered containers.

possible, keep the vegetables from touching the boiling water and pack them loosely enough for the steam to circulate well.

If you boil vegetables, use as little water as possible, since water removes nutrients. To retain the most vitamin C, bring the water to a boil before you put in the vegetables. Remove vegetables from the water while they are still firm; otherwise, they may become soft from overcooking. The cooking water, which contains vitamins and minerals, can be used as the base for soups or sauces.

You can also stir-fry vegetables in a wok or heavy skillet, using one or two tablespoons of vegetable or olive oil. The vegetables should be cut uniformly so that they all cook at about the same rate. Before adding the vegetables, heat the oil so that it is very hot but not smoking. Add soft, thin vegetables like spinach or chard at the last moment — they will cook in less than a minute.

When cooking frozen vegetables, do not automatically follow the package directions. For firmer, better-tasting vegetables, try reducing the suggested cooking time. Serve cooked vegetables immediately: The longer they sit, the more their vitamin content decreases.

The recipes that follow offer an interesting and satisfying variety of ways to cook and serve vegetables. Many of them provide hearty, filling main courses without using meat — allowing you to put nutritional punch into a meal with relatively few calories.

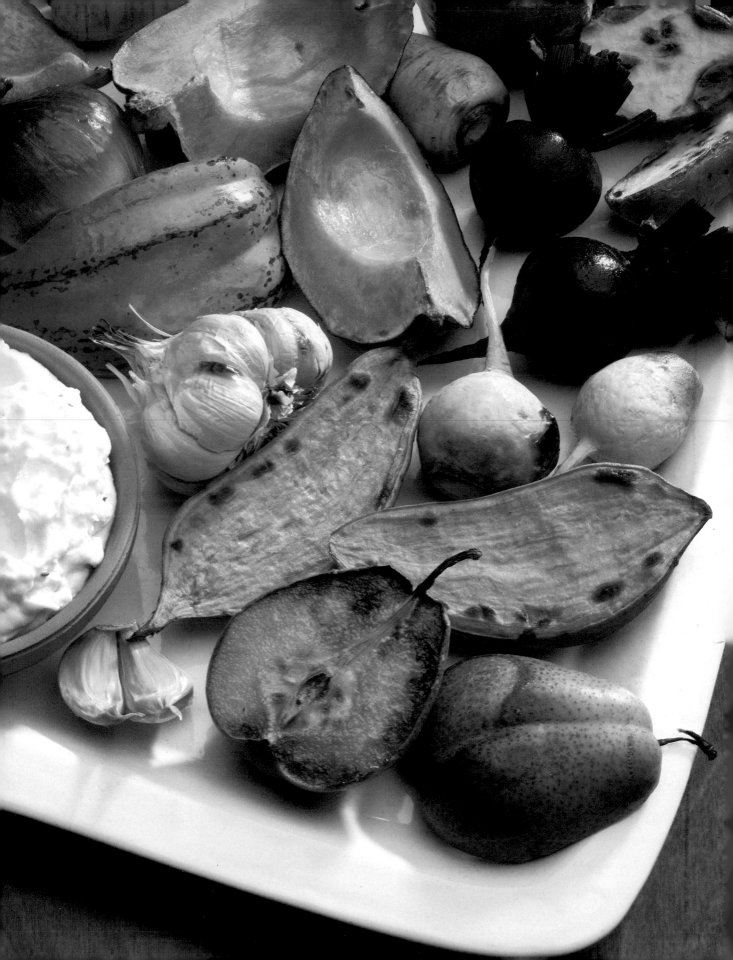

ROASTED VEGETABLES WITH GARLIC SAUCE

Recent cardiovascular studies suggest that a diet that includes plenty of onions may increase your supply of beneficial HDL cholesterol. Each serving of this hearty main dish includes a whole onion.

2 small new potatoes, or 1 medium-size baking potato
1 medium-size sweet potato
1 small acorn squash
2 medium-size turnips, trimmed
2 medium-size beets, stems trimmed to 1 inch
2 medium-size parsnips, trimmed
1 medium-size pear
1/2 teaspoon olive oil
2 medium-size red onions
2 heads of garlic
1/2 teaspoon salt
3/4 cup nonbutterfat sour dressing
Black pepper

CALORIES	564
66% Carbohydrate	100 g
9% Protein	13 g
25% Fat	17 g
CALCIUM	229 mg
IRON	4 mg
SODIUM	709 mg

Preheat the oven to 500° F. Wash the vegetables and the pear. Halve the potatoes lengthwise, quarter the squash and halve the pear; brush the cut sides lightly with oil. Leave the turnips, beets, parsnips and onions whole. Peel the outer layer of skin from the garlic heads but do not peel or separate the cloves. Arrange the vegetables and pear halves in a roasting pan, placing the cut vegetables and the pear cut side up, and sprinkle with salt. Roast about 30 minutes, or until the vegetables are tender when pierced with a fork. Remove the garlic and cover the pan with foil to keep warm.

For the sauce, separate the garlic cloves and squeeze the cloves out of their skins into a bowl; discard the skins. Using a fork, mash the garlic and mix in the sour dressing and pepper to taste. Arrange the vegetables and pear on a platter and serve the garlic sauce on the side. Makes 2 servings

TARRAGON TOMATO JUICE

Unlike soft drinks, which contain mostly water and sugar, this spicy low-calorie drink contributes vitamins A and C and niacin, a B vitamin your body needs in order to utilize carbohydrates for energy.

8 medium-size ripe tomatoes, peeled, seeded and coarsely chopped (4 cups)
1/2 teaspoon salt
1/4 teaspoon pepper
3/4 cup balsamic or other red wine vinegar
1 tablespoon finely chopped fresh tarragon

Place the tomatoes in a large nonreactive saucepan and cook over low heat about 5 minutes, or until the tomatoes begin to break down and render their juices. Transfer the tomatoes to a food processor or blender and purée, then transfer the purée to a pitcher and add the salt, pepper and vinegar. Refrigerate the juice until well chilled. Just before serving, stir in the tarragon.

Makes 4 servings

Note: If fresh tarragon is unavailable, substitute fresh basil, dill or parsley.

CALORIES	42
79% Carbohydrate	10 g
14% Protein	2 g
7% Fat	.4 g
CALCIUM	18 mg
IRON	1 mg
SODIUM	296 mg

I ceberg lettuce may be the best-selling lettuce, but darker varieties of lettuce, like Romaine, contain more vitamins and minerals. Romaine lettuce has more than five times as much beta carotene (which the body turns into vitamin A) and three times as much vitamin C as iceberg. Romaine contains more than three times as much calcium as iceberg and more than twice as much iron.

The nutritional analyses accompanying these recipes provide nutrient values per serving, unless otherwise indicated.

◁ *Roasted Vegetables with Garlic Sauce*

CHARD AND POTATO RAVIOLI

Chard, sometimes called Swiss chard, contains substantial calcium, and a serving of this ravioli supplies almost half the calcium you need daily. Drinking fortified lowfat milk with this dish will enhance your body's absorption of the calcium from the vegetables.

CALORIES	**481**
61% Carbohydrate	**74 g**
17% Protein	**21 g**
22% Fat	**12 g**
CALCIUM	**374 mg**
IRON	**5 mg**
SODIUM	**512 mg**

1 large baking potato (10 ounces)
1/2 pound chard or spinach leaves, finely chopped
1 tablespoon unsalted butter
3/4 cup chopped onion
4 large mushrooms, chopped
1 ounce prosciutto, finely chopped
1/4 teaspoon salt
1 1/4 teaspoons coarsely ground pepper
10-ounce package wonton wrappers

1 whole clove
1 small onion, halved
1 garlic clove, crushed and peeled
1 1/2 cups evaporated skimmed milk
2 tablespoons whole milk
1 slice firm white bread, trimmed of crusts and torn into small pieces
2 bay leaves
1/4 cup toasted walnuts, chopped
3 tablespoons chopped fresh parsley

Bring a small saucepan and a large pot of water to a boil. Cook the potato in the saucepan 20 minutes. Meanwhile, blanch the chard in the large pot 1 minute; drain, cool under cold water and squeeze out the excess moisture. In a large skillet, melt the butter over medium-high heat. Add the chopped onions and mushrooms and cook 3 minutes, or until the onions are slightly softened. Add the chard and continue cooking about 5 minutes, or until the chard is tender. Add the prosciutto, salt and 1/4 teaspoon of pepper, and toss. When the potato is cooked and cool enough to handle, peel and crumble it and add it to the chard.

Line a baking sheet with a kitchen towel; set aside. Using a pastry brush or your fingertip, moisten the edge of a wonton wrapper with water. Place a heaping teaspoon of the potato-chard filling on one side of the wrapper, fold over and press firmly to seal *(opposite)*. Make 48 ravioli in this fashion. Place the ravioli on the towel-lined baking sheet, cover with another towel and wrap in plastic wrap. Set aside until the sauce is made.

For the sauce, bring enough water to a boil in the bottom of a double boiler so that the boiling water will not touch the top pan. Insert the whole clove into one of the onion halves. Place the onion halves, garlic, evaporated and whole milk, bread and bay leaves in the top pan and cook over boiling water 20 minutes. Remove and discard the onion, garlic and bay leaves. Transfer the mixture to a food processor or blender and purée, then set aside.

Bring a large pot of water to a boil. Drop 12 ravioli into the boiling water and cook about 5 minutes, or until al dente. Cook the remaining ravioli in the same fashion. Drain and divide the ravioli among 4 plates. Briefly reheat the sauce and pour it over the ravioli. Sprinkle with the walnuts, parsley and the remaining teaspoon of black pepper.

Makes 4 servings

Note: Wonton wrappers or skins, sometimes called gyoza wrappers, are small thin disks of pasta dough. They are sold in Chinese grocery stores and in the refrigerated sections of many supermarkets.

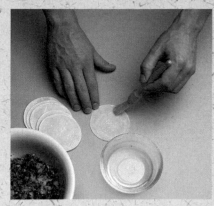 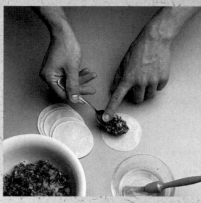 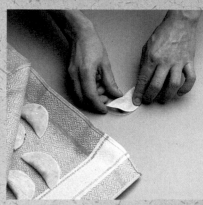

Separate the wonton wrappers. Using a small pastry brush and working with one wonton wrapper at a time, moisten the edges of the wrapper with water.

Place a heaping teaspoon of the potato-chard filling on one side of the moistened wonton wrapper. Do not overfill, or the wrapper will not stay sealed.

Fold the wrapper over the filling and press firmly to seal. Place the ravioli on a towel-lined baking sheet and cover with a second towel to keep moist.

SPINACH-STUFFED BAKED POTATOES

Frying potatoes adds fat and destroys vitamins. Stuffing baked potatoes, as you do here, with spinach, tomatoes and cheese adds fiber, calcium and potassium, as well as vitamins A and C and niacin.

CALORIES	287
71% Carbohydrate	54 g
15% Protein	11 g
14% Fat	5 g
CALCIUM	200 mg
IRON	6 mg
SODIUM	960 mg

2 large baking potatoes (1 1/4 pounds total weight)
5 ounces spinach, stems removed
1 1/2 teaspoons butter
1/4 cup skim milk
1/2 cup chopped tomato

2 scallions, chopped
Pinch of nutmeg
3/4 teaspoon salt
1/2 teaspoon pepper
1 tablespoon grated Gruyère cheese

Preheat the oven to 450° F. Bake the potatoes about 1 hour, or until they are tender when pierced. Meanwhile, steam the spinach about 3 minutes. Drain, squeeze dry and coarsely chop the spinach; set aside. Split the potatoes lengthwise and scoop out the pulp, leaving a 1/4-inch-thick shell. Mash the pulp with the butter and milk, then add the spinach, tomato, scallions, nutmeg, salt and pepper, and mix well. Spoon the mixture into the potato shells and sprinkle with Gruyère. Bake the potatoes 6 to 8 minutes, or until the stuffing is heated through and the cheese is lightly browned. Makes 2 servings

COLLARD, CABBAGE AND SWEET POTATO SAUTE

The collard greens in this main dish are one of the best vegetable sources of calcium. A cup of collards supplies just as much calcium as a cup of milk.

CALORIES	115
68% Carbohydrate	21 g
12% Protein	4 g
20% Fat	3 g
CALCIUM	180 mg
IRON	1 mg
SODIUM	206 mg

1 pound collard greens, leaves and tender stems only, chopped, or 10-ounce package frozen collard greens, thawed
1/2 cup low-sodium chicken stock
2 teaspoons olive oil
1 small onion, finely diced
1/2 large celery rib, finely diced
1 small carrot, finely diced
1 large sweet potato, finely diced

1/8 teaspoon red pepper flakes
1 tablespoon sugar
1/4 teaspoon salt
1/4 teaspoon pepper
2 garlic cloves, chopped
1 teaspoon tomato paste
2 cups shredded cabbage (about 1/4 pound)
3/4 teaspoon chopped fresh rosemary

Combine the collards and stock in a large nonstick skillet, cover and cook over medium heat, tossing occasionally, about 20 minutes, or until tender; drain and transfer to a large bowl. Set aside. If using frozen collards, drain and squeeze dry. Heat the oil in the same skillet over medium-high heat. Add the onion, celery, carrot, sweet potato and red pepper flakes and cook, stirring occasionally, about 20 minutes, or until the vegetables soften and begin to brown. Add the sugar, salt and pepper, and cook another 3 to 4 minutes, or until the vegetables are well browned. Add the garlic and tomato paste and cook another minute, or just until the garlic is fragrant. Add the cabbage, rosemary and collards and cook, tossing, until the cabbage wilts slightly and the collards are heated through. Makes 4 servings

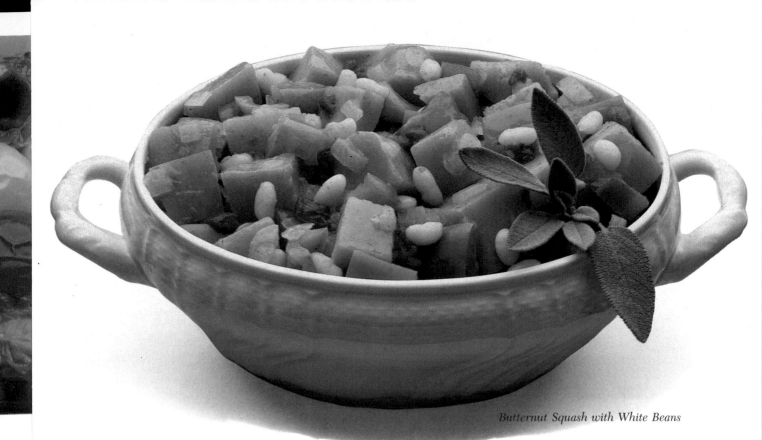

Butternut Squash with White Beans

BUTTERNUT SQUASH WITH WHITE BEANS

The butternut squash in this side dish supplies a sizable amount of niacin.

1 1/2 teaspoons olive oil
1 cup coarsely diced onion
1 large garlic clove, peeled and
   minced
1 cup diced tomato
1 cup diced green bell pepper
1 pound butternut squash,
   peeled and cut into 1-inch cubes

1/4 teaspoon sage
1/8 teaspoon allspice
Pinch of Cayenne pepper
1 bay leaf
1/4 teaspoon salt
1/3 cup low-sodium chicken stock
1/2 cup cooked white beans
Splash of vinegar

In a medium-size heavy-gauge saucepan, heat the oil over medium heat. Add the onion and half of the garlic, and sauté for 1 minute. Reduce the heat slightly, cover the pan and cook 5 minutes, or until the onions are soft. Add the tomato and green pepper and cook another 2 minutes. Add the squash, sage, allspice, Cayenne, bay leaf, salt and stock, and cook, covered, over medium heat 15 minutes. Add the beans and cook, uncovered, 5 minutes, or until the squash is soft but not mushy. Increase the heat to high and cook just until any remaining liquid evaporates. Add the remaining garlic and the vinegar, and toss to combine. Serve immediately. Makes 3 servings

CALORIES	158
71% Carbohydrate	31 g
13% Protein	6 g
16% Fat	3 g
CALCIUM	105 mg
IRON	3 mg
SODIUM	200 mg

CALORIES	592
73% Carbohydrate	94 g
16% Protein	22 g
11% Fat	6 g
CALCIUM	301 mg
IRON	8 mg
SODIUM	459 mg

A salad bar should offer more than just nutritious food. It should be equipped with an overhanging cover that prevents dust and contaminants from settling on the food. Items that need refrigeration should sit in enough ice to keep them cold. And the bar should be monitored by an employee who makes sure that customers do not touch food with their hands or use serving utensils that have dropped on the floor. Otherwise, foods at the salad bar, especially high-protein foods like eggs, meat, poultry and fish, can become contaminated with infectious organisms.

PASTA AND VEGETABLES IN MISO BROTH

Bok choy is one of the leafy green vegetables high in beta carotene, which your body converts into vitamin A.

1 cup low-sodium chicken stock
1 cup sake (Japanese rice wine)
8 medium-size mushrooms, sliced
4 scallions, finely chopped
6 parsley sprigs
2 ounces fresh ginger, thinly sliced
2 garlic cloves, thinly sliced
1/2 cup julienned turnip
1 large carrot, julienned
1/2 medium-size head bok choy, stems thinly sliced and leaves shredded, separated (2 1/4 cups total)

2 teaspoons Japanese rice-wine vinegar
Pinch of Cayenne pepper
1/2 teaspoon Oriental sesame oil
1 tablespoon reduced-sodium soy sauce
1 1/2 tablespoons miso
1 bunch watercress, stems trimmed to 1/2 inch
6 ounces spaghetti, cooked and drained
1 tablespoon sesame seeds
1 tablespoon toasted nori, cut into thin strips

In a medium-size saucepan, combine the stock, sake, mushrooms, scallions, parsley, ginger, garlic and 2 cups of water, and bring to a boil. Reduce the heat and simmer the broth 30 minutes. Strain the broth into a bowl, discard the solids and return the broth to the pan (you should have about 3 cups). Add the turnip, carrot and bok choy stems and simmer about 2 minutes. Add the vinegar, Cayenne, sesame oil and soy sauce. Transfer 1/2 cup of the broth to a small bowl, stir in the miso and return the mixture to the pan. Add the bok choy leaves, watercress and spaghetti, remove the pan from the heat, and stir to wilt the greens. Ladle the mixture into 2 soup bowls and sprinkle with sesame seeds and nori. Makes 2 servings

Note: Nori, a Japanese dried seaweed, is rich in calcium and iron. To toast it, hold it with tongs over high heat for about 5 seconds, or just until crisped.

PENNE WITH RED PEPPER SAUCE

This colorful pasta dinner dish provides plenty of carbohydrates, iron and vitamin C.

2 large red bell peppers
1/4 pound green beans
6 ounces penne or other pasta
1 tablespoon olive oil
2 medium shallots, finely chopped
2 garlic cloves, minced
1/2 cup white wine
1/2 cup low-sodium chicken stock
1 medium-size tomato, chopped

2 small leeks, washed and cut crosswise into 1/4-inch pieces
1 large yellow bell pepper, cut into 1/4-inch-wide strips
1 teaspoon chopped fresh rosemary
1/2 teaspoon salt
1/4 teaspoon black pepper
2 tablespoons goat cheese, crumbled (1 ounce)

Preheat the broiler. Broil the red peppers about 5 inches from the heat, turning frequently, until they are charred all over. Place the peppers in a paper bag and let them steam 15 minutes. Meanwhile, bring a medium-size saucepan and a large pot of water to a boil. Blanch the green beans in the saucepan about 5 minutes, or until just tender; drain and cool under cold water. Cook the pasta in the large pot of boiling water until al dente; drain and set aside. Peel, seed and chop the red peppers, place in a blender and purée.

Heat the oil in a large nonstick skillet over medium heat. Add the shallots and garlic, and sauté 1 minute. Cover and cook another 4 minutes, or until the shallots are soft. Add the wine and stock, bring to a gentle boil and cook about 3 minutes, or until the liquid is reduced to about 3/4 cup. Add the tomato, leeks and yellow pepper, and simmer about 3 minutes, or until the liquid is reduced to about 1/2 cup. Add the green beans, red pepper purée, rosemary, salt, pepper and half of the goat cheese, and simmer 1 minute. Toss the sauce with the pasta, add the remaining cheese and toss again.

Makes 2 servings

CALORIES	541
73% Carbohydrate	101 g
12% Protein	16 g
15% Fat	9 g
CALCIUM	150 mg
IRON	8 mg
SODIUM	602 mg

Penne with Red Pepper Sauce

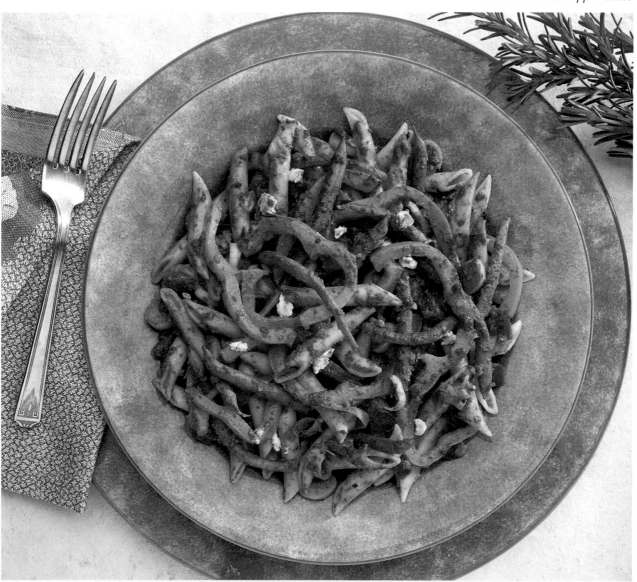

SPICY POTATO AND CHICKPEA SALAD

Besides being a good source of complex carbohydrates, vitamin C and fiber, potatoes are an outstanding source of potassium.

CALORIES	308
60% Carbohydrate	47 g
11% Protein	9 g
29% Fat	10 g
CALCIUM	93 mg
IRON	4 mg
SODIUM	596 mg

1 anchovy fillet, drained
1 tablespoon olive oil
1/2 cup chopped onion
2 garlic cloves, chopped
2 tablespoons white wine
3 tablespoons low-sodium chicken stock
2 tablespoons sherry vinegar or red wine vinegar
1/4 teaspoon salt
1 teaspoon ground cumin
1/4 teaspoon paprika
1/8 teaspoon ground cloves
Pinch of Cayenne pepper

2/3 cup canned chickpeas, rinsed and drained
4 medium-size potatoes, boiled and cut into 1-inch pieces
1 large red bell pepper, roasted (see page 40), peeled and cut into 1/4-inch-wide strips
4 pitted black olives, halved
1/4 cup chopped scallions
1 1/2 tablespoons chopped fresh parsley
1 1/2 tablespoons chopped fresh coriander

In a medium-size skillet, heat the anchovy in the oil over medium heat, stirring with a wooden spoon, until the anchovy disintegrates and the oil is hot. Add the onion and garlic and cook 1 minute, tossing to coat with oil, then cover and cook 4 to 5 minutes, or until the onion is soft. Add the wine and boil gently until almost all of the liquid has evaporated. Add the stock, vinegar, salt,

Spicy Potato and Chickpea Salad

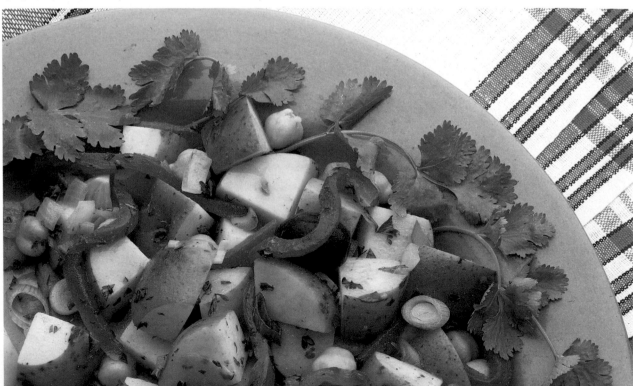

cumin, paprika, cloves and Cayenne, and simmer another 2 minutes. Remove the skillet from the heat, add the chickpeas and potatoes, and toss gently. Add the pepper strips, olives, scallions, parsley and coriander and toss again. Serve at room temperature.   Makes 2 servings

GRILLED EGGPLANT SANDWICH

Eggplant absorbs a lot of fat when it is fried. Grilling it with a topping of onions helps keep it from drying out while cooking, so it requires only a minimal amount of oil.

CALORIES	202
54% Carbohydrate	28 g
13% Protein	7 g
33% Fat	8 g
CALCIUM	81 mg
IRON	2 mg
SODIUM	165 mg

3 large plum tomatoes, peeled, seeded and chopped (2 cups)
1 cup thinly sliced mushrooms
1 tablespoon balsamic or other red wine vinegar
1/4 teaspoon fennel seeds
Eight 1/4-inch-thick eggplant slices (about 1/2 pound)

1/2 medium-size red onion, thinly sliced
2 teaspoons olive oil
Black pepper
1 English muffin
2 tablespoons grated fontina cheese

For the sauce, combine the tomatoes, mushrooms, vinegar and fennel seeds in a small nonreactive saucepan. Cook, covered, over medium heat 10 minutes, or until the juices are rendered. Uncover the pan and cook another 15 minutes, or until the sauce is thickened and reduced to about 1 cup.

Meanwhile, preheat the oven to 500° F. Place the eggplant slices on a baking sheet, top with onion slices and brush with 1 teaspoon of the oil. Sprinkle with salt, and pepper to taste, and bake 4 minutes. Brush the onions and eggplant with the remaining oil and bake another 3 to 4 minutes, or until the vegetables are soft.

Preheat the broiler. Split and toast the English muffin. Spread the muffin halves with half of the tomato sauce and place 4 onion-topped eggplant slices on each half. Top with the remaining sauce and sprinkle with cheese. Broil the sandwiches about a minute, or until the cheese melts.   Makes 2 servings

CARROT BREAD PUDDING

Carrots are a rich source of beta carotene. The beta carotene content of carrots increases for up to 20 weeks in cold storage after harvesting.

CALORIES	230
81% Carbohydrate	48 g
7% Protein	4 g
12% Fat	3 g
CALCIUM	64 mg
IRON	2 mg
SODIUM	89 mg

1 1/2 cups grated carrots
1 1/4 cups fine dry bread crumbs
2 tablespoons currants
3/4 teaspoon nutmeg

1/4 teaspoon ground cloves
4 large eggs
1 1/2 cups brown sugar
1/2 teaspoon vanilla

Preheat the oven to 325° F. In a large bowl, combine the grated carrots, bread crumbs, currants, nutmeg and cloves, and stir well. In another large bowl, using an electric mixer, beat the eggs and brown sugar for about 5 minutes, or until the mixture is thick and smooth. Beat in the vanilla. Fold the egg mixture gently into the carrot mixture and pour into a 1 1/2-quart casserole. Bake the pudding 35 minutes, or until the center is set.   Makes 8 servings

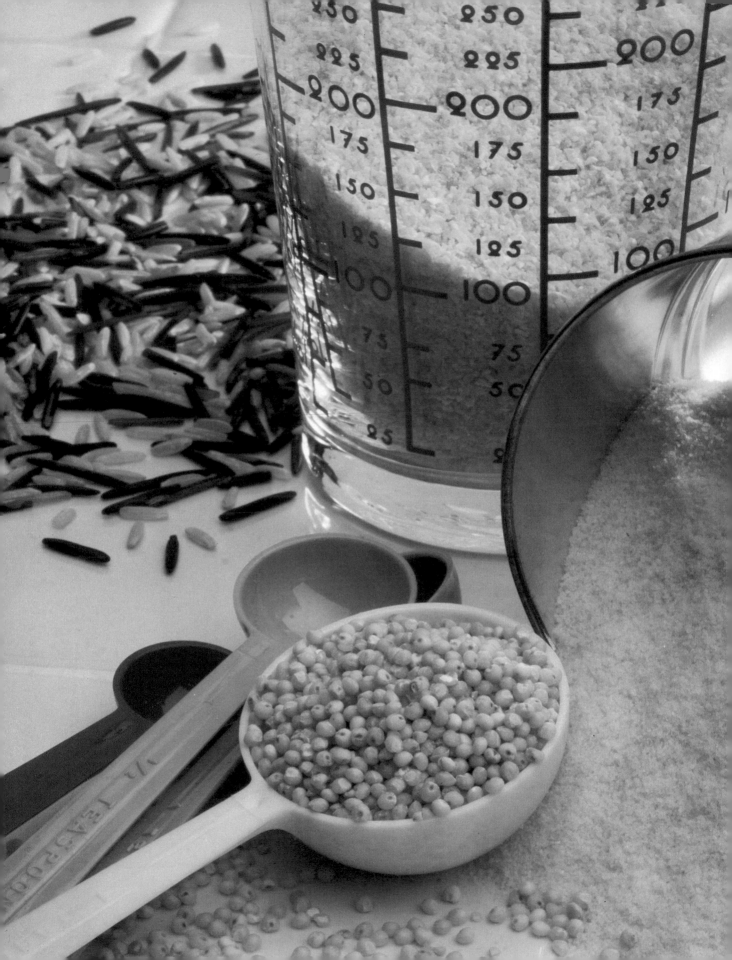

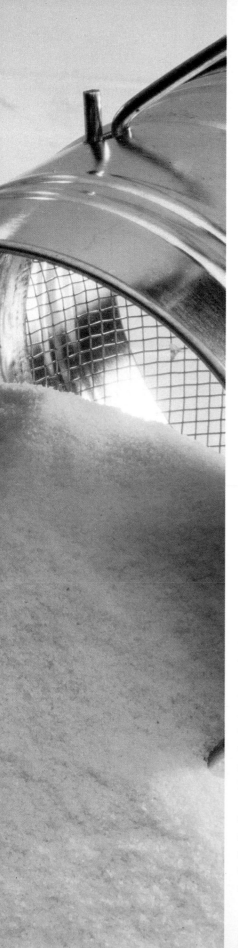

Grains

High in carbohydrates, a superb source of fiber and suitable for a wide range of cooking methods

The case for making grains part of a healthy diet is simple: They are the principal source of complex carbohydrates, which means they provide energy without an excess of fattening calories. Half a cup of cooked pasta or rice, for example, contains 20 grams of complex carbohydrates with no simple sugars. In addition, most grains are rich in B vitamins. Wheat, the most widely consumed grain, also supplies protein and every vitamin and mineral except vitamins A, B_{12} and C and the mineral iodine. Oats contain all seven of the B vitamins and vitamin E. And all of the grains, when refined only minimally, are high in fiber.

Rice, corn, wheat, oats, barley, millet and most other grains share a similar structure. The core consists of a protein-rich germ, or embryo, and a surrounding endosperm, which is a concentrated source of complex carbohydrates, vitamins and minerals. Together these form the seed. A layer of fiber-rich bran encases the seed, and the whole is enclosed in an inedible hull, or husk.

BARLEY *Boil, uncovered, for 45 minutes in an unlimited amount of water, or simmer, covered, for 45 minutes, using 2 parts water to 1 part barley.*

BROWN RICE *Simmer, covered, for 45 minutes, using 2 parts water to 1 part rice.*

COUSCOUS *Steep, uncovered, for 40 minutes, using 1 part boiling water to 2 parts couscous, or steam, covered, for 1 hour.*

CRACKED WHEAT (BULGUR) *Steep, uncovered, for 30 minutes, using 1 part boiling water to 2 parts cracked wheat; or simmer, covered, for 40 minutes, using 2 parts water to 1 part cracked wheat; or steam, covered, for 1 hour.*

GRITS *Steep, uncovered, for 30 minutes, using 1 part boiling water to 2 parts grits, or simmer, covered, for 15 minutes, using 2 parts water to 1 part grits.*

KASHA *Simmer, covered, for 15 minutes, using 2 1/2 parts water to 1 part kasha.*

Unfortunately, most of us eat grains in their least nutritious state: as white rice; as breads, rolls, cakes and pasta made from highly refined flour; and as overprocessed breakfast cereal. These products lack both the bran and the germ, which are typically removed in the milling process (but are retained in whole-grain products). Refined white wheat flour, for example, loses up to 80 percent of the vitamins and minerals present in the whole kernel, and it retains only seven percent of the fiber. Some vitamins are replaced by fortification but none of the fiber is. Similar losses occur when other grains are refined and when the kernels of such grains as rice and barley are polished. When brown rice is polished to produce white rice, the grain loses almost half of its riboflavin and more than half of its niacin.

Studies show that people living in countries where unrefined whole grains comprise a significant portion of the diet have lower levels of certain intestinal and bowel diseases than in Western industrialized countries. Much of this difference is attributed to the fiber in unrefined grains. A lack of dietary fiber has been linked to constipation. And research has proved that a diet high in the water-soluble fiber contained in oats can hold down blood cholesterol levels.

In their least refined but still edible state, with only the husks removed, whole grains are called groats or berries. When the berries are crushed, they are said to be "cracked." Examples of cracked whole grains are cracked wheat and cracked corn (which is known as hominy and has the germ removed). Some grains, such as the wheat product called bulgur, are steamed after being cracked. Others, like rolled oats or oat flakes, are steamed and then crushed by rollers. Such refining methods preserve more nutrients than the process of refining grain into bleached flour.

Since most of us consume more grains in our breads than anywhere else, the easiest way to get more nutrition from grain products is to eat whole-wheat, cracked-wheat or oatmeal bread instead of white bread. You can also substitute whole-grain breakfast cereals like oatmeal for refined cereal, choose brown rice instead of white rice, and eat the less common grains such as barley, millet and kasha. Another way to consume more whole grains is to sprinkle wheat bran, wheat germ, rice bran or rice germ on cereals, yogurt and fruit. You can also mix these grains into the dough for such baked goods as muffins and quickbreads.

Breads and cereals are the most common grain dishes, but the high carbohydrate content of grains makes them a good basis for main dishes as well. If eaten alone, though, grains do not supply all of the protein you need, since the protein in grains lacks some of the essential amino acids. To get complete protein in a meal based on grains, you should add legumes, nuts, dairy products or a small amount of meat containing the missing amino acids. If the ingredients in a recipe do not accomplish this, round out the meal with a glass of milk, some cheese, a dish of yogurt for dessert, or another source of complete protein.

Cooking grains yourself is the best way to ensure that you will eat

Buying and Storing Guide

◆ Always buy whole-grain products from a store that has a rapid turnover of merchandise. Whole grains have more nutritive value than heavily refined grains but a shorter shelf life because the oils in whole grains can turn rancid. Avoid whole grains that look or smell dusty or old.

◆ When buying commercially made whole-grain breads, always check to see that the first ingredient listed on the package is whole wheat or another whole grain; this indicates that it is the primary ingredient. Do not be misled by the color of the bread or by its name. A dark bread can be made from refined grains that are darkened with molasses. And a bread labeled "whole wheat" may actually contain a minimal amount of the whole grain.

◆ Whole-wheat flour, the most widely used whole grain, and brown rice should always be kept in the refrigerator, where they can be stored safely for six to eight months. Both white flour and white rice, if stored in a cool, dry place, will last indefinitely.

◆ Grain products other than whole-wheat flour and rice will usually keep for up to three months if refrigerated. But they must be stored in tight containers to prevent them from absorbing moisture. Frozen grains can be stored for three to six months.

them in their most nutritious, least refined state. Grains lend themselves to a variety of cooking and baking techniques. Some baked goods, like corn tortillas (made from cornmeal) and oatcakes (made from oatmeal), use whole grains. But most conventional recipes for bread and pasta call for refined white flour. Whole-grain flours can usually be substituted for white flour or used in combination with it. If you do use white flour, make sure it is unbleached.

Because they are dry, grains must be cooked in water to become tender. They can be boiled, simmered, steamed or steeped to achieve different effects. Boiling yields the fluffiest, driest grains. To prevent lumping, make sure the water is boiling hard, then slowly stir in the grains. Steaming is suitable for tender cracked grains such as millet, cracked wheat and bulgur. However, these grains should be left uncovered while steaming and tossed regularly to prevent clumping. Steeping grains — soaking the kernels in water that has first been brought to a boil — imparts a chewy texture to cracked wheat and bulgur. No matter how you prepare them, grains will triple or quadruple in volume as they absorb water.

Cooking times for the grains featured in this chapter are listed in the box on the opposite page. (As a rule of thumb, the less refined the grain, the longer it takes to cook.) The recipes that follow offer a variety of ways to use grains and should encourage you to include more of them in your diet. Indeed, grains can and should be a part of every meal, not only as side dishes or breads, but as appetizers, main courses and desserts.

GRITS WITH DRIED APPLE AND BACON

CALORIES	205
61% Carbohydrate	31 g
13% Protein	7 g
26% Fat	6 g
CALCIUM	65 mg
IRON	2 mg
SODIUM	464 mg

Hominy grits, like all grains, lack complete protein. But combining the grits with an animal product like bacon — which has complete protein — enables your body to make full use of all the amino acids that are present in the grain.

1 1/2 cups apple juice
1 teaspoon salt
3/4 cup hominy (corn) grits
3 strips bacon

1 tablespoon unsalted butter
1 cup skim milk
2 eggs
1/3 cup finely chopped dried apple

In a medium-size saucepan, bring the apple juice and 2 cups of water to a boil. Add the salt and slowly stir in the grits. Reduce the heat, cover the pan and simmer 20 minutes, stirring frequently.

Preheat the oven to 350° F. Fry the bacon until crisp. Crumble the bacon and set aside. Add the butter, milk and eggs to the cooked grits and stir well. Stir in the apple and crumbled bacon. Turn the grits into a shallow 9-inch baking dish and bake 1 hour and 10 minutes, or until the top is golden and beginning to brown.   Makes 6 servings

Kasha-Potato Pancakes

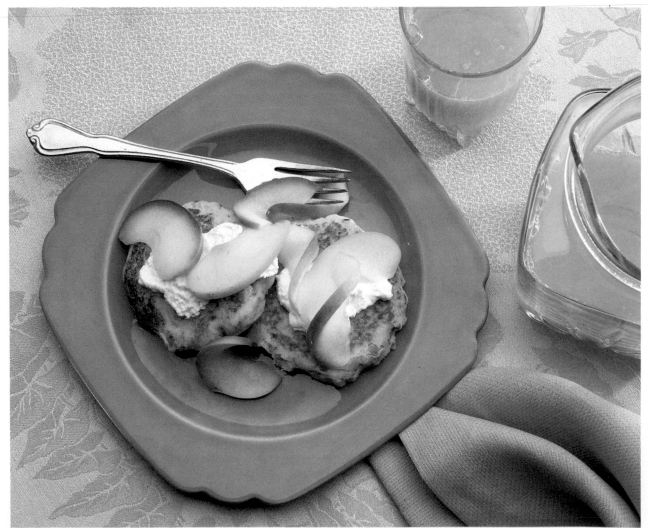

RYE APPLESAUCE MUFFINS

When buying rye flour, choose as dark a variety as you can find — the darker flour is less refined and contains more nutrients.

Vegetable cooking spray
1/3 cup rye flakes
2/3 cup rye flour
1/2 cup unbleached all-purpose
 flour
1/2 cup whole-wheat flour
1/2 teaspoon salt
1 tablespoon baking powder
1 teaspoon ground ginger

1/2 teaspoon ground cardamom
1 cup chunky applesauce
1 large egg, lightly beaten
3/4 cup plus 2 tablespoons skim
 milk
1/4 cup honey
3 tablespoons vegetable oil
1 teaspoon grated lemon peel

Preheat the oven to 400° F. Spray 12 muffin tin cups with cooking spray. Sift together the dry ingredients onto a sheet of wax paper, then resift into a large bowl. In a medium-size bowl combine the applesauce, egg, milk, honey, oil and lemon peel. Pour the applesauce mixture over the dry ingredients and stir just until combined. Do not overmix. Divide the batter equally among the 12 muffin tin cups and bake about 20 minutes, or until a toothpick inserted in the center of a muffin comes out clean.   Makes 12 muffins

CALORIES per muffin	142
63% Carbohydrate	23 g
8% Protein	3 g
29% Fat	5 g
CALCIUM	84 mg
IRON	1 mg
SODIUM	214 mg

KASHA-POTATO PANCAKES

Buckwheat groats, also known as kasha, are an excellent lowfat, low-calorie protein source, with half as much protein per pound as beef.

1/3 cup kasha (whole groats)
4 medium-size potatoes, boiled,
 peeled and mashed (2 cups)
1 tablespoon butter
1/2 teaspoon salt
1/4 teaspoon pepper

1/2 teaspoon caraway seeds
1 Golden Delicious apple
2 tablespoons apple cider
1 large egg, separated
Vegetable cooking spray
8 teaspoons lowfat cottage cheese

Bring 2/3 cup of water to a boil in a small saucepan. Add the kasha, cover and simmer 15 minutes, or until all the liquid has been absorbed. In a large bowl combine the kasha, potatoes, butter, salt, pepper and caraway seeds. Stir until blended. Refrigerate the mixture about 2 hours, or until well chilled.

Meanwhile, core and thinly slice the apple. Cook the apple slices in the cider in a small saucepan, covered, over medium heat 3 to 5 minutes, or until softened but still somewhat firm; remove the pan from the heat and set aside. Add the egg yolk to the chilled kasha mixture and stir to combine. In a large bowl, using an electric mixer, beat the egg white until stiff peaks form. Fold the egg white into the kasha mixture. Spray a nonstick skillet with cooking spray and heat it over medium heat. Using half of the kasha mixture, make four 3-inch pancakes. Cook the pancakes about 4 minutes on each side, or until golden brown, then transfer them to a platter and cover with foil to keep warm. Make 4 more pancakes in the same fashion. Divide the pancakes among 4 plates and top each serving with 2 teaspoons of cottage cheese and one fourth of the apple slices.   Makes 4 servings

CALORIES	171
62% Carbohydrate	27 g
11% Protein	5 g
27% Fat	5 g
CALCIUM	35 mg
IRON	1 mg
SODIUM	363 mg

VEGETABLE SOUP

This light vegetable soup is thickened with cornmeal. The soup contains a large amount of vitamin A in its carrots, zucchini, yellow squash and broccoli, as well as protein in its cornmeal and cheese.

2 teaspoons olive oil

1 1/2 cups chopped onion

1/2 cup diced carrot

1 cup diced red bell pepper

2/3 cup diced celery

2 garlic cloves, minced

1/3 cup thinly sliced zucchini

1/3 cup thinly sliced yellow squash

2/3 cup broccoli florets

1/3 cup yellow cornmeal

1/4 cup thinly sliced scallions

2 teaspoons chopped fresh coriander

2 tablespoons grated Parmesan

In a large saucepan, heat the oil over medium heat. Add the onion, carrot, bell pepper, celery and garlic, reduce the heat to low and cook about 10 minutes, or until the onions are soft. Increase the heat to high and add 6 cups of water. Bring the soup to a boil and add the zucchini, yellow squash and broccoli. Reduce the heat and simmer about 7 minutes, or until the broccoli is tender. Increase the heat to high and bring the soup to a rolling boil. Slowly pour in the cornmeal, whisking constantly. Continue whisking about 1 minute, or until the soup thickens. Remove the pan from the heat and ladle the soup into 4 bowls. Sprinkle each serving with scallions, coriander and Parmesan.

Makes 4 servings

CALORIES	123
62% Carbohydrate	20 g
13% Protein	4 g
25% Fat	4 g
CALCIUM	83 mg
IRON	1 mg
SODIUM	78 mg

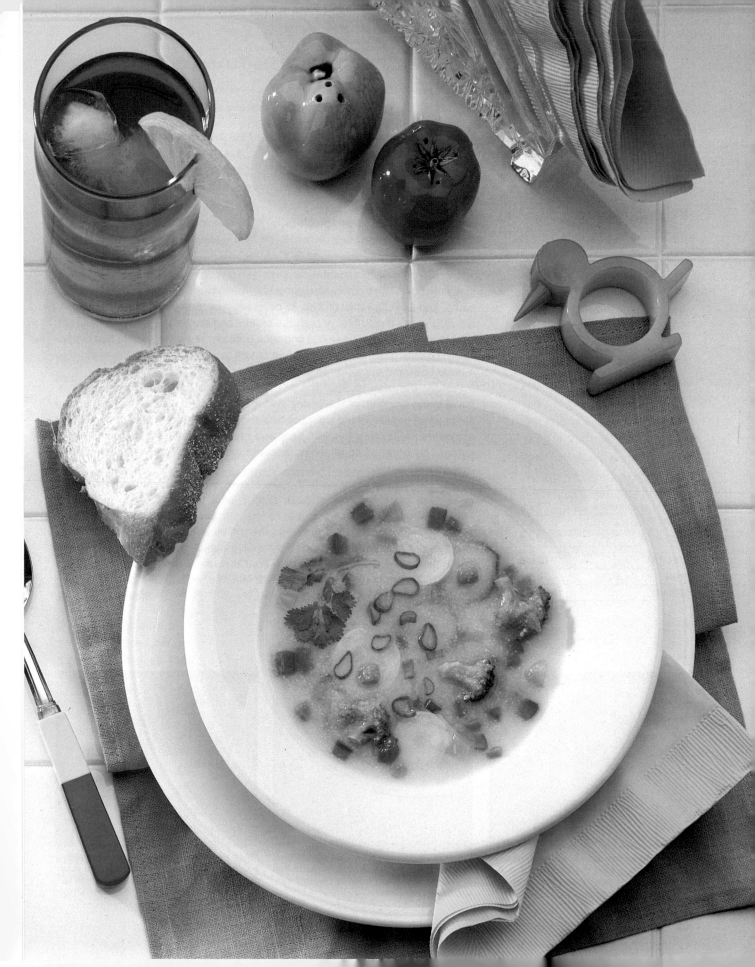

BROWN RICE SUSHI ROLLS

CALORIES	392
66% Carbohydrate	66 g
11% Protein	11 g
23% Fat	10 g
CALCIUM	135 mg
IRON	4 mg
SODIUM	732 mg

Both brown rice and tofu are good dietary sources of iron. A serving of this sushi contains more than 20 percent of the iron men need daily.

1 tablespoon plus 2 teaspoons Japanese rice-wine vinegar
1 tablespoon sugar
1/4 teaspoon salt
2 cups cooked short-grain brown rice (3/4 cup raw), at room temperature (see Note)
1 1/4 teaspoons Oriental sesame oil
1 tablespoon plus 1 teaspoon reduced-sodium soy sauce
1/2 teaspoon sherry
1/4 teaspoon grated fresh ginger
3 1/2 ounces firm tofu, cut into 1/2 × 3 1/2-inch strips
1/4 teaspoon grated orange peel
Two 7 × 8-inch sheets nori (Japanese dried seaweed), or 2 large cabbage leaves
10 fresh basil leaves
1/4 red bell pepper, cut into 1/4-inch-wide strips
1 scallion, julienned
1/4 avocado, peeled and cut into 1/2-inch-thick slices
1 carrot, finely julienned

In a small saucepan, heat the vinegar, sugar and salt until the sugar dissolves. Place the rice in a medium-size bowl and toss it lightly with the vinegar mixture and 1 teaspoon of oil. In a small bowl, combine the remaining oil, 1 teaspoon of soy sauce, the sherry and ginger. Add the tofu and toss to combine; set

Brown Rice Sushi Rolls

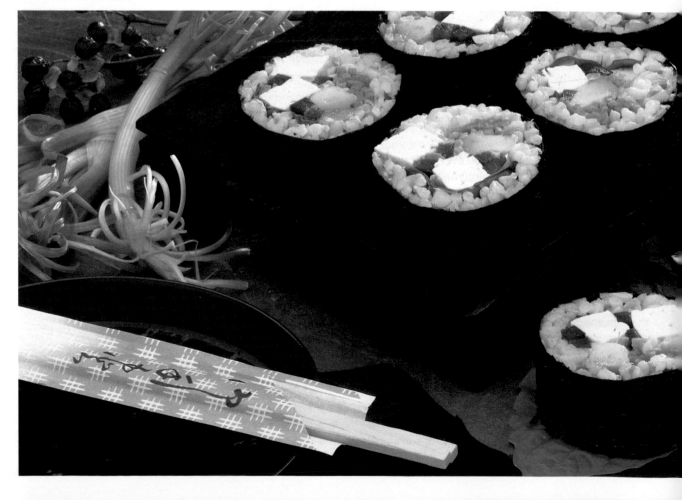

aside. Combine the orange peel and remaining soy sauce in a small bowl; set aside. If using cabbage leaves, bring a large pot of water to a boil. Blanch the leaves 15 seconds, or just until wilted. Cool the leaves under cold water, pat dry with paper towels and cut out the tough center ribs.

Place a sheet of nori, shiny side down, or a cabbage leaf, on a clean dish-cloth so that a short side of the nori or leaf is toward you. Spread 1 cup of rice evenly over the nori, leaving 1/2-inch borders at the top and bottom. Using half of the ingredients, arrange the filling on the rice in the following manner: About one third of the way from the top, lay the basil leaves in a row. Place the tofu strips horizontally on top of the basil. Arrange the bell pepper strips horizontally below the tofu, then add rows of scallion strips, avocado slices and carrot strips below the peppers. Pick up the near edge of the dishcloth and the nori and begin rolling it tightly away from you, holding the filling in place with your fingers. When the edges of the nori meet, peel back the dishcloth so it does not catch in the roll. When the roll is completely formed, squeeze it gently; the nori should stick to itself. Moisten it slightly if it does not stick. Set the roll aside for a few minutes, then carefully remove the dishcloth, transfer the roll to a cutting board and cut it crosswise into 8 slices. Make a second sushi roll in the same fashion. Makes 2 servings

Note: If the rice has been refrigerated, it will have lost the necessary sticki-ness. To restore the stickiness, place the rice and 1/2 cup of water in a small saucepan. Bring it to a simmer, cover the pan tightly, reduce the heat to low and steam the rice 5 minutes. Set aside to cool slightly.

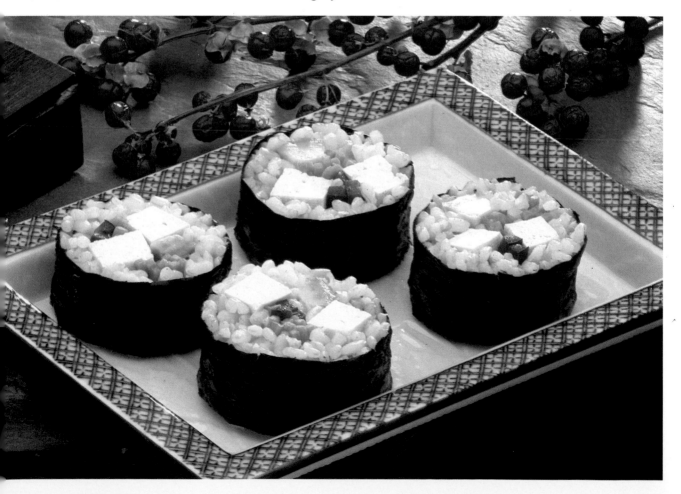

CALORIES	330
69% Carbohydrate	57 g
18% Protein	15 g
13% Fat	5 g
CALCIUM	418 mg
IRON	4 mg
SODIUM	193 mg

D*espite their wholesome image, most granola bars are not much better for you than regular candy bars. Granola bars usually contain as much saturated fat as a pat of butter, and they often derive more than 70 percent of their calories from sugar and fat. The meager amounts of oats and nuts in a granola bar give it only a slim nutritional edge over the standard candy bar.*

CALORIES	140
77% Carbohydrate	29 g
13% Protein	5 g
10% Fat	2 g
CALCIUM	42 mg
IRON	1 mg
SODIUM	44 mg

BROWN RICE PUDDING

Studies at Cornell University indicate that women who exercise have an increased need for riboflavin, a B vitamin that the cells must have to release energy. A serving of this custard-like rice pudding supplies more than 25 percent of your daily requirement of riboflavin.

Vegetable cooking spray
4 large eggs
1 3/4 cups skim milk
1 3/4 cups evaporated skimmed milk
1/4 cup nonfat dry milk
1/2 cup maple syrup

2 cups cooked brown rice (3/4 cup raw)
1/2 vanilla bean, split
1/4 cup chopped crystallized ginger
3/4 teaspoon grated lemon peel
1/8 teaspoon ground cinnamon
1/8 teaspoon ground nutmeg

Preheat the oven to 350° F. Spray a 2-quart baking dish with cooking spray. Bring a large pot of water to a boil. Meanwhile, in a large bowl, combine the eggs, liquid and dry milks and maple syrup. Stir in the rice, vanilla bean, ginger and lemon peel. Pour the mixture into the baking dish, place the dish in a large baking pan and add enough boiling water to the pan to reach halfway up the side of the baking dish. Bake the pudding 50 minutes, or until the custard-like part is just set. Sprinkle the pudding with cinnamon and nutmeg and let cool to lukewarm. Stir the pudding before serving to blend the rice with the custard. Remove and discard the vanilla bean.   Makes 6 servings

BULGUR AND FIG SOUFFLES

Refined wheat products, even when enriched, are low in fiber, zinc and copper — all of which are abundant in less refined grains like bulgur.

1/4 teaspoon unsalted butter
6 dried black figs, halved
1 cup orange juice, preferably freshly squeezed
1 cinnamon stick

1 cup cooked bulgur (1/3 cup raw)
1 teaspoon grated orange peel
3 egg whites
2 tablespoons nonbutterfat sour dressing

Lightly butter four 6-ounce ovenproof ramekins; set aside. In a medium-size nonreactive saucepan, combine the figs, orange juice, cinnamon stick and 1/2 cup of water. Simmer over low heat 20 minutes, or until the figs are soft.

Preheat the oven to 400° F. Using a slotted spoon, transfer the cooked figs to a food processor or blender; reserve the poaching liquid. Add the bulgur to the figs and process about 1 minute, or until the figs are puréed. Transfer the mixture to a medium-size bowl and set aside to cool slightly. Cook the poaching liquid over high heat about 4 minutes, or until it is reduced to about 1/3 cup. Remove and discard the cinnamon stick. Stir the liquid into the fig mixture, then stir in the orange peel; set aside to cool.

Meanwhile, in a large bowl, using an electric mixer, beat the egg whites until they hold stiff peaks. Fold one third of the whites into the fig mixture to lighten it, then carefully fold in the remaining egg whites. Divide the mixture equally among the ramekins and bake in the center of the oven 13 minutes, or until the tops of the soufflés are puffed and crusty. Top each soufflé with 1 1/2 teaspoons of sour dressing and serve immediately.   Makes 4 servings

UPSIDE-DOWN APPLE TART

While this dessert recipe contains some saturated fat from butter, most of the fat is from corn oil, which is primarily unsaturated.

1 teaspoon unsalted butter	3/4 teaspoon baking powder
3 tablespoons sugar	1/8 teaspoon baking soda
1 large Granny Smith apple, cored and cut into 1/4-inch-thick slices	2 tablespoons nonbutterfat sour dressing
1/2 teaspoon ground cinnamon	1 egg
Pinch of ground nutmeg	1/2 tablespoon corn oil
1/2 cup yellow cornmeal	

CALORIES	115
66% Carbohydrate	20 g
7% Protein	2 g
27% Fat	4 g
CALCIUM	35 mg
IRON	1 mg
SODIUM	83 mg

Preheat the oven to 400° F. In a 10-inch ovenproof skillet, melt the butter over medium heat. Add 2 tablespoons of sugar and cook 30 seconds. Stir in 1 tablespoon of water. Arrange the apple slices in a circle in the skillet, overlapping them slightly if necessary. Increase the heat to high and cook about 3 minutes, or until the outer edges of the apples are dark brown. Remove the skillet from the heat.

In a medium-size bowl, combine the dry ingredients, including the remaining tablespoon of sugar; set aside. In a small bowl, mix the sour dressing and 2 tablespoons of water. Add the egg and beat lightly with a fork. Add this mixture to the dry ingredients, then add the oil and stir briefly with a wooden spoon just until combined. Do not overmix. Pour the batter over the apples in the skillet and bake on the upper rack of the oven 8 to 10 minutes, or until the crust is cooked through. Remove the skillet from the oven and place it over high heat briefly, shaking to loosen the tart, then carefully invert the tart onto a platter.

Makes 6 servings

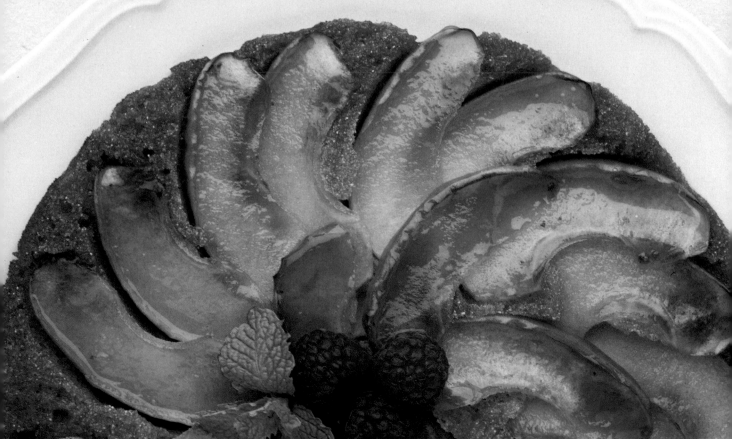

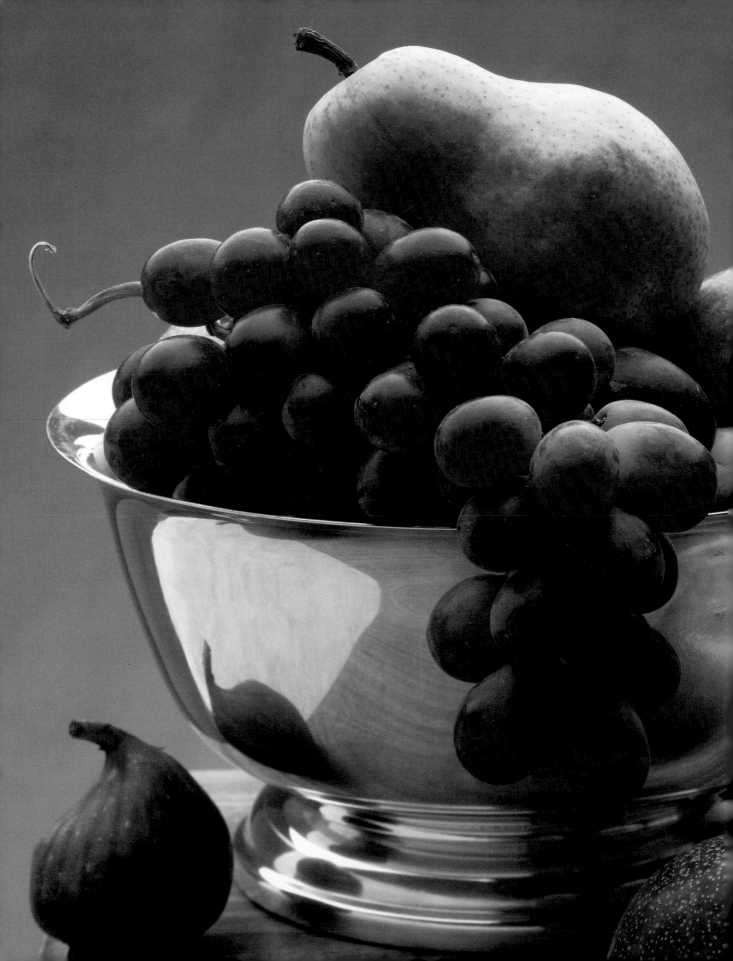

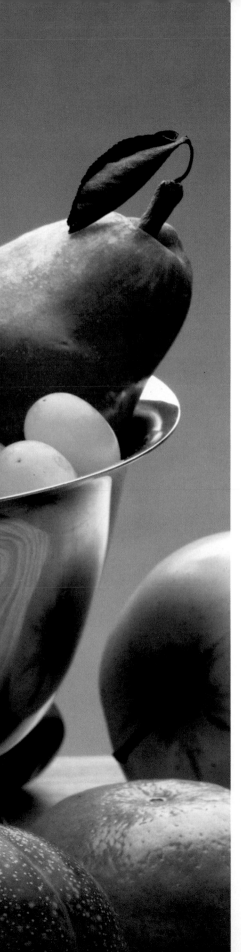

CHAPTER FOUR

Fruits

*Sweet-tasting with few calories
and plenty of vitamin C*

The chief appeal of many fruits is that they taste sweet yet are relatively low in calories. What keeps their calorie content down is water — most fruits are 80 to 95 percent water, which also makes them juicy and thirst-quenching. Moreover, since they typically contain a great deal of fiber, fruits can add satisfying bulk to your diet. Besides water and fiber, fruits provide fructose· (natural fruit sugar), starches (complex carbohydrates), a very small amount of protein and a healthy assortment of vitamins and minerals. Except for avocados, olives and coconuts, fruits usually contain only a trace of fat and no artery-clogging cholesterol. Raw fruits make nutritious, low-calorie desserts or snacks, unlike most baked goods, which are loaded with saturated fat and refined sugar.

Fruits, along with vegetables, supply virtually all the vitamin C in the American diet — 92 percent — but only nine percent of the calories. Vitamin C, or ascorbic acid, is crucial for maintaining healthy blood vessels, capillaries, teeth and gums. It also helps your body absorb iron. And because this vitamin is used to make collagen, the fabric of your connective tissue, it aids in the healing of cuts and burns.

Citrus fruits, including oranges, grapefruit, pineapples, lemons and limes, are the most dependable year-round sources of vitamin C. Just one orange fulfills your daily requirement of this vitamin — 60 milligrams. Half a cup of strawberries also provides your daily requirement of vitamin C and more fiber than a slice of whole-wheat bread, but fewer than 40 calories. Such exotic fruits as papaya, kiwi and guava are also high in ascorbic acid.

Some fruits are rich sources of beta carotene, which your body converts to vitamin A. This vitamin promotes good vision and helps form and maintain healthy skin as well as the linings of the throat, lungs and urinary tract. Recent studies have shown that beta carotene may also protect against some types of cancer. Yellow and orange fruits like apricots, peaches, mangoes and cantaloupes tend to be the highest in beta carotene. Thus, half a cantaloupe — with only 60 calories — supplies you with more than enough vitamin A for a whole day, while a honeydew has less than two percent of the daily requirement. (The cantaloupe also provides a day's worth of vitamin C.)

One of the most important minerals found in fruits is potassium, essential for maintaining normal blood pressure, heartbeat and muscle contraction. Bananas, pears and oranges are among the best fruit sources of potassium. Fruits also provide some iron (in blackberries, raspberries, strawberries, dried apricots, prunes, dates and figs) and even small amounts of calcium (in dates, figs and oranges).

Raw fresh fruits are generally more nutritious than frozen or canned varieties. Most fresh fruits suffer minimal loss of vitamin C, beta carotene and other nutrients during storage. While vegetables can lose a quarter of their vitamin C after one day in the refrigerator, many whole fruits retain this vitamin for seven to 10 weeks. Vitamin C in fruit is destroyed by exposure to air, however; whole fruits retain more of this vitamin than fruits that have been sliced, cooked or otherwise processed.

The peel plays a vital role in supplying and preserving nutrients. For example, peeling an apple can lower its modest vitamin C content by 25 percent. If you do peel a piece of fruit because a recipe requires it, peel it as thinly as possible to minimize nutrient loss, and do not peel it until shortly before using it. To minimize the loss of vitamins, do not slice fruits very thinly. The thinner and smaller the slices or pieces are, the more surface area you expose to the oxygen in the air, which destroys vitamins.

Drinking fruit juices, either store-bought or made in your own juicer, is another good way to incorporate fruits into your diet. Their vitamins and minerals make them healthy substitutes for soft drinks, which contain only sugar, water, preservatives and artificial flavoring. Freshly squeezed citrus juice or juice freshly made from frozen concentrate, if refrigerated, remains high in vitamin C for at least a week. Apple, cranberry, grape, pineapple and prune juices have very

Buying and Storing Guide

Fruits do not have to look perfect to be good. Some quite edible citrus fruits, for example, have superficial patches and scars. But, as a rule, you should look for relatively unblemished fruits and avoid those that have obvious insect damage or are wrinkled, overripe or otherwise injured. Buy fruits that are at least beginning to ripen, rather than unripe ones; the fruits should be firm rather than hard and in many cases should smell faintly sweet. Whenever possible, buy fruits in season, when their quality is at its peak.

In general, berries should be bought ripe enough to eat immediately. Blueberries can usually be stored up to two weeks in the refrigerator in a covered container. Strawberries should have their green caps intact until just before they are served; this preserves their vitamin C. Raspberries are best eaten within 24 hours of ripening.

Pick out grapefruit that feel the densest and smoothest. All grapefruit increase in vitamin C content as they ripen, but pink grapefruit have substantially more beta carotene than the white variety. Oranges should feel heavy and firm; spongy oranges will not be as juicy. Both grapefruit and oranges last longest when they are refrigerated.

It is usually best to purchase bananas that are slightly green and let them ripen at room temperature. You can accelerate the ripening process by putting the bananas in a paper bag. Once they are ripe, store them in the refrigerator.

little vitamin C, unless they have been processed by a manufacturer who has fortified them. Even then, it has been shown that vitamin C breaks down much more quickly in these juices than in orange or grapefruit juice.

Dried fruits — such as apples, apricots, dates, figs, peaches, prunes and raisins — have more calories than an equivalent amount of the fresh varieties because drying reduces the water content by about 75 percent, thus increasing the caloric density. Although you should not snack on dried fruits too often, particularly if you are watching your weight, they are richer in various nutrients, particularly potassium and iron, and higher in fiber than many other snack foods. And sulfuring processes, which are often used in drying to keep the fruits' colors from darkening, help preserve vitamins A and C. For anyone who is sensitive to sulfur or who wants to avoid preservatives, health-food stores stock preservative-free dried fruits. Some people dry their own fruits at home.

Using fruits to add sweetness to prepared dishes is one of the best ways to eliminate high-fat, high-sugar foods from your diet while improving your vitamin and mineral intake. The following recipes combine fruits with a wide variety of foods. As your palate becomes accustomed to more fruits and less refined sugar, you should find it easier to cut back on the amount of sugar in your diet.

CALORIES	318
71% Carbohydrate	56 g
13% Protein	10 g
16% Fat	6 g
CALCIUM	166 mg
IRON	2 mg
SODIUM	432 mg

BLUEBERRY CORNMEAL PANCAKES

A cup of fresh blueberries contains about one third of your daily requirement of vitamin C. Adding the berries — fresh or frozen — to these cornmeal pancakes also gives you a good deal of fiber.

1 1/4 cups unbleached
  all-purpose flour
1 cup yellow or white cornmeal
1 1/2 teaspoons baking soda
1 teaspoon baking powder
Pinch of salt

2 1/4 cups buttermilk
2 eggs, separated, plus 1 egg white
3 tablespoons dark brown sugar
2 cups fresh or frozen blueberries
1 tablespoon vegetable oil

In a small bowl, stir together the flour, cornmeal, baking soda, baking powder and salt; set aside. In a large bowl, whisk together the buttermilk, egg yolks and sugar; set aside. In another large bowl, using an electric mixer, beat the egg whites until stiff peaks form. Add the dry ingredients to the buttermilk mixture and stir until blended, then gently fold in the egg whites. Stir in the blueberries. Heat 1/2 teaspoon of oil in a large nonstick skillet over medium heat. Using 1/4 cup of batter for each pancake, make 4 pancakes, cooking them about 4 minutes on each side or until golden brown. Make 5 more batches of pancakes in the same fashion, adding 1/2 teaspoon of oil to the skillet before cooking each batch.   Makes 6 servings

*H*ard candies are worse for your teeth than large helpings of ice cream or cake. The reason: Hard candies stay in your mouth longer and expose your teeth to the harmful, cavity-causing effects of sugar for a prolonged period. Similarly, although fruit juices are better for you than soft drinks, the sugar in both can be bad for your teeth if you do not brush them within a few hours of drinking these beverages.

ORANGE-PRUNE MUFFINS

Dried fruits like prunes have more carbohydrates and calories per ounce than raw fruits because their sugar content remains the same after the water has been removed. With only 20 calories, however, a prune still has 15 calories less than a pat of butter — and virtually no fat.

12 prunes, cut into eighths
1/4 cup orange juice
3/4 cup buttermilk
1 tablespoon grated orange peel
1 3/4 cups unbleached all-purpose
  flour
1 teaspoon baking powder
1/2 teaspoon baking soda

1/2 teaspoon salt
1/4 cup vegetable oil
2 tablespoons molasses
2 tablespoons dark brown sugar
1 egg
1 cup cooked cracked wheat (1/3
  cup raw)

CALORIES per muffin	174
64% Carbohydrate	28 g
8% Protein	4 g
28% Fat	6 g
CALCIUM	55 mg
IRON	1 mg
SODIUM	185 mg

Preheat the oven to 400° F. Lightly spray 12 muffin tin cups with cooking spray or line them with paper liners. Cook the prunes and orange juice in a small nonreactive saucepan over medium-low heat 4 minutes, or until almost all the liquid has evaporated. Remove from the heat and stir in the buttermilk and orange peel; set aside. In a medium-size bowl, combine the flour, baking powder, baking soda and salt, and make a well in the center. In another medium-size bowl, combine the oil, molasses, sugar and egg, and mix until blended. Add the prunes and cracked wheat, and mix until blended. Pour the mixture into the well in the dry ingredients and stir just until combined. Divide the batter among the muffin tin cups and bake 20 minutes, or until the muffins are browned on top and firm to the touch.   Makes 12 muffins

MUESLI

Dried fruit is a fair source of iron. One serving of this muesli provides more than 15 percent of the RDA of iron for adult women.

2 cups rolled oats
1 cup skim milk
1/4 cup currants or raisins
1/4 cup apple juice
2 tablespoons honey
1 cup plain lowfat yogurt

1/4 cup minced dried apricots
1/2 cup minced dried apples
1/4 cup ground hazelnuts
1/4 cup brown sugar
2 tangerines, peeled, sectioned
  and seeded

Place the oats in a medium-size bowl, pour in the milk and stir well. In a small bowl, combine the currants and apple juice. Set aside both mixtures for 30 minutes.

   Stir the honey into the yogurt; set aside. Add the currants and apple juice, the dried fruit, hazelnuts and sugar to the oats, and stir well. Divide the muesli among 4 bowls and top each serving with 1/4 cup of yogurt and some tangerine sections.

Makes 4 servings

CALORIES	394
74% Carbohydrate	75 g
12% Protein	12 g
14% Fat	6 g
CALCIUM	234 mg
IRON	3 mg
SODIUM	89 mg

DUCK SALAD WITH GINGERED PEARS

In some people high blood pressure may be exacerbated by consuming too much sodium and too little potassium. Fruits like pears, which contain 65 times more potassium than sodium, can improve your sodium/potassium ratio.

CALORIES	298
55% Carbohydrate	42 g
17% Protein	13 g
28% Fat	9 g
CALCIUM	44 mg
IRON	4 mg
SODIUM	52 mg

1/4 cup sherry
1 1/2 teaspoons grated fresh
  ginger
4 medium-size Anjou pears,
  peeled, halved and cored
3 tablespoons olive oil
2 tablespoons Japanese rice-wine
  vinegar
1 teaspoon Dijon-style mustard

Pinch of black pepper
3/4 pound asparagus, trimmed
6 ounces fedelini or spaghettini
1 cup julienned red bell pepper
1/2 cup julienned scallion
1/2 pound skinless, boneless duck
  breast (2 breasts)
Small head red leaf lettuce

Combine the sherry, ginger and 1/4 cup of water in a medium-size nonreactive saucepan. Add the pears, cover and bring to a boil. Reduce the heat and simmer, stirring occasionally, 7 to 10 minutes, or until the pears are fork-ten-

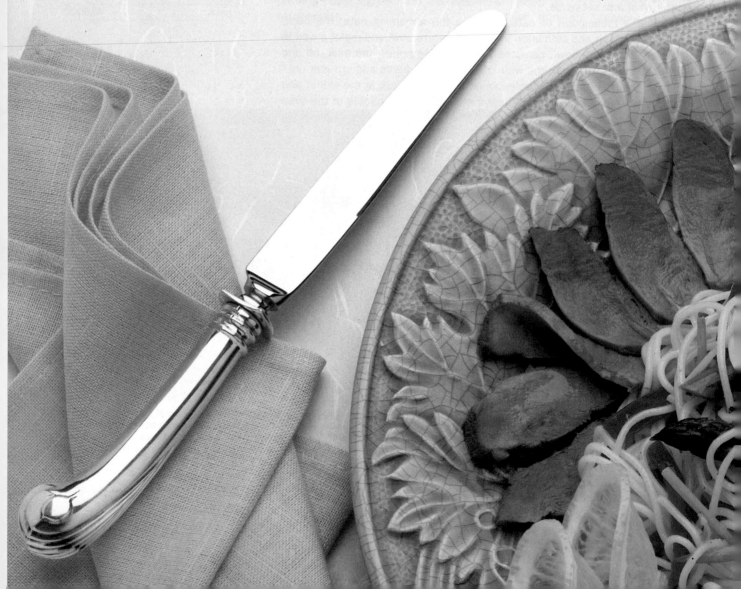

der. Drain the pears, reserving the liquid for the vinaigrette. Transfer the pears to a bowl and refrigerate until well chilled. For the vinaigrette, in a small bowl combine 1/3 cup of the reserved cooking liquid with the oil, vinegar, mustard and pepper; set aside.

Bring a large pot of water to a boil. Cut off and reserve the asparagus tips. Cut the remaining stalks diagonally into 2-inch lengths and blanch 2 minutes. Add the tips and cook another minute. Using a slotted spoon, transfer the cooked asparagus to a colander; reserve the boiling water. Cool the asparagus under cold running water, transfer to a large bowl and set aside. Cook the pasta in the boiling water according to the package directions until al dente. Drain the pasta and add it to the asparagus. Add the bell pepper, scallion and half of the vinaigrette, and toss to combine. Let stand 1 hour.

Meanwhile, sauté the duck breasts in a medium-size nonstick skillet over medium heat 3 to 4 minutes on each side, or until the juices run pink when the meat is pierced with a sharp knife. Remove the skillet from the heat and let the cooked duck rest 5 minutes, then cut it on the diagonal into thin slices.

To serve, line 6 dinner plates with lettuce leaves. Cut the pears into thin slices. Mound some of the pasta-vegetable mixture in the center of each plate, then arrange the pear and duck breast slices around it.   Makes 6 servings

CRANBERRY-SPICE SYRUP

CALORIES	33
98% Carbohydrate	9 g
1% Protein	.1 g
1% Fat	.04 g
CALCIUM	8 mg
IRON	.1 mg
SODIUM	2 mg

After hot-weather exercise, fruit-flavored drinks made from this concentrate and the two recipes that follow will replenish some of the fluids and electrolytes you lose in perspiration.

1 cup unsweetened cranberry juice
Pinch of ground ginger
Pinch of ground cinnamon
Pinch of ground allspice
Pinch of ground cloves
Two 1/4-inch-thick orange slices, unpeeled

Combine all the ingredients in a nonreactive saucepan, bring to a boil over medium-high heat and cook at a slow boil for 10 minutes. Remove the orange slices and pour the syrup into a jar or bottle. Cover and refrigerate.

For a Cranberry-Spice Fizz, place 3 tablespoons of syrup in a tall glass and add 8 ounces of seltzer; for a Cranberry-Spice Toddy, place 3 tablespoons of syrup in a mug and add 8 ounces of boiling water and a cinnamon stick. The syrup will keep for about a month in the refrigerator.   Makes 5 servings

BLUEBERRY-VANILLA SYRUP

CALORIES	57
91% Carbohydrate	14 g
4% Protein	.6 g
5% Fat	.4 g
CALCIUM	6 mg
IRON	.2 mg
SODIUM	6 mg

1 pint fresh blueberries
1-inch piece of vanilla bean, split

Place the blueberries in a food processor or blender and process to a purée. Transfer the purée to a bowl, cover and let stand overnight in a cool place (not the refrigerator). Place a cheesecloth-lined strainer over a medium-size bowl and strain the purée, squeezing out as much juice as possible; you should

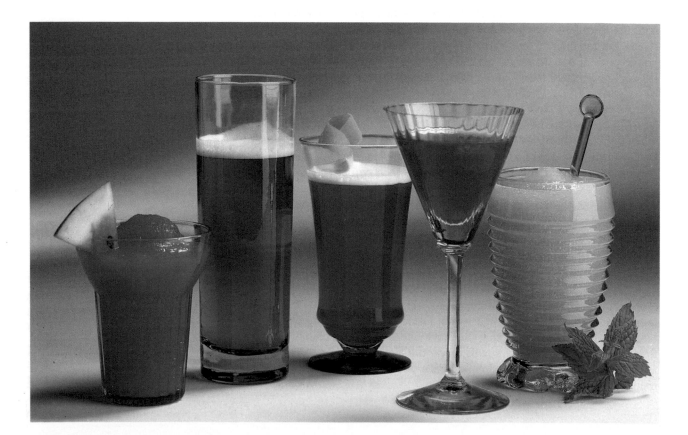

have about 1/2 cup. Place the juice and the vanilla bean in a nonreactive saucepan and bring to a boil over medium-high heat. Cook at a slow boil for 10 minutes. Pour the liquid into a jar or bottle and cover tightly.

For drinks, follow the directions for Cranberry-Spice Syrup *(above)*. You can also use the Blueberry-Vanilla Syrup on pancakes.

Makes 3 servings

RASPBERRY SYRUP

1/2 pint fresh raspberries

Follow the directions for Blueberry-Vanilla Syrup *(above)*.

Makes 2 servings

CALORIES	64
85% Carbohydrate	15 g
6% Protein	2 g
9% Fat	1 g
CALCIUM	28 mg
IRON	1 mg
SODIUM	0 mg

WATERMELON CRUSH

This unusual, refreshing watermelon drink gives you 25 percent of the RDA for vitamin A and 50 percent of the RDA for vitamin C, as well as potassium from the banana.

1 1/4 pounds watermelon (weighed with rind)

1/2 medium-size banana
4 ice cubes

Scoop the flesh of the watermelon into a large bowl and crush it with a potato masher. Cover the bowl and refrigerate overnight. Place a cheesecloth-lined strainer over a medium-size bowl and strain the watermelon, squeezing out as much juice as possible; you should have about 3/4 cup. Combine the juice, banana and ice in a blender and process until the mixture is slushy; pour into a chilled glass.

Makes 1 serving

CALORIES	153
86% Carbohydrate	36 g
6% Protein	3 g
8% Fat	2 g
CALCIUM	27 mg
IRON	1 mg
SODIUM	7 mg

HONEYDEW SLUSH

"Slush" or "snow" drinks made with sugary syrups are nutritionally empty snacks, but this fruit-based refresher is rich in vitamin C and potassium, and contains small amounts of some B vitamins and minerals.

1 large honeydew melon (about 2 1/4 pounds)

3 ice cubes

To prepare the honeydew juice, halve the melon and remove and discard the seeds. Follow the directions for Watermelon Crush *(above)*. Combine the juice and ice cubes in a blender and process until slushy. Pour into a chilled glass.

Makes 1 serving

CALORIES	194
93% Carbohydrate	51 g
5% Protein	3 g
2% Fat	1 g
CALCIUM	33 mg
IRON	.4 mg
SODIUM	55 mg

◁ *Watermelon Crush; Blueberry-Vanilla, Cranberry-Spice and Raspberry Fizzes; Honeydew Slush*

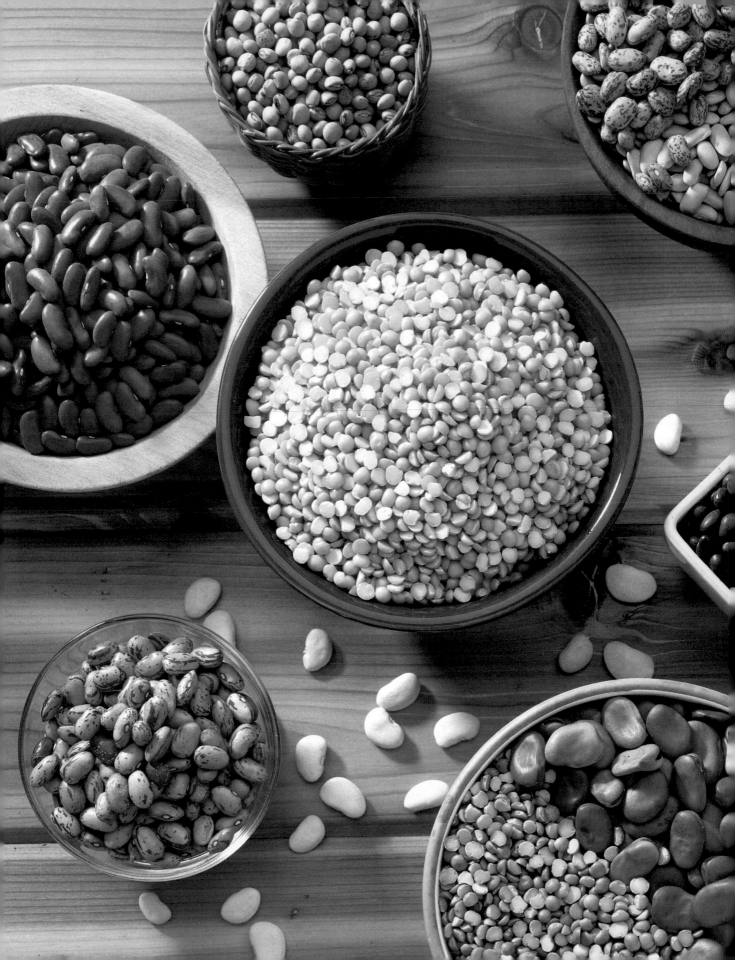

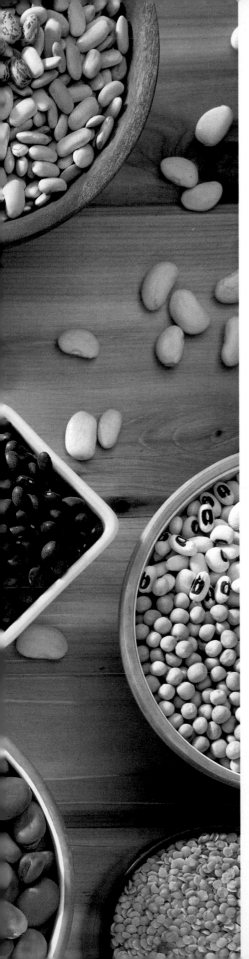

CHAPTER FIVE

Legumes

The best plant source of protein

Although they are high in a number of nutrients, legumes — which include beans, peas, lentils and peanuts — are especially rich in protein. On average, these pod-borne seeds when mature (or dried) contain about 22 percent protein, more than any other plant food. And unlike animal-derived protein, the protein in legumes is free of cholesterol and usually low in fat. Consequently, the protein you get from most legumes comes in a low-calorie package compared to meat. A filling half-cup serving of cooked legumes averages only 120 calories; a lean six-ounce hamburger supplies approximately 280 calories.

Legumes are also high in energy-providing complex carbohydrates, in B vitamins (particularly B_6 and thiamin), and in the minerals iron, zinc, magnesium and copper. A half-cup serving of most cooked legumes provides 12 percent of the daily Recommended Dietary Allowance (RDA) of iron for women and 20 percent for men, as well as up to 10 percent of the RDA of zinc for both men and women. Moreover, because legumes are low in sodium and high in potassium, they are especially good for people who have high blood pressure. And sprouted legumes, such as alfalfa sprouts and the mung-bean sprouts often used in Chinese dishes, also provide a great deal of vitamin C.

Averaging about nine grams of fiber per half-cup serving, legumes provide the highest concentration of fiber of any plant food. Recent studies have shown that the water-soluble fiber in legumes may actually lower cholesterol levels in the blood — and thus the risk of cardiovascular disease — by binding with dietary cholesterol and then carrying it out of the body. Preliminary evidence suggests that this cholesterol-lowering effect may be long-lasting. In addition, legumes can help those who are watching their weight. Because they contain so much indigestible fiber, legumes fill you up with relatively few calories.

Although most legumes are incomplete proteins — that is, they lack one or more of the essential amino acids the body needs to utilize protein fully — it is easy to complete their protein by eating them with a small amount of grains, dairy products, eggs, poultry or meat. You can even eat the complementary foods a few hours after consuming the legumes and still receive the benefits of the full protein. Most of the recipes that follow show how to combine legumes with other foods so that they can serve as the main protein source in a meal.

The way legumes are cooked is important, particularly if you are subject to intestinal gas and bloating. Flatulence is a condition that occurs when complex sugars produce gas as they break down in the lower intestine. It is sometimes a problem for those who are not used to eating legumes regularly, though many people have no trouble at all. By preparing dried legumes in a three-step process of cleaning, soaking and cooking, you can minimize this difficulty. The first step, cleaning, is important because dried beans, packaged or loose, often contain bits of sediment. Be sure to pick over the beans carefully, then immerse them briefly in water. Remove and discard any beans that float to the top and then rinse the remainder again in cold water.

Soaking, the second step, is required because most dried beans have to be rehydrated after the ripening and drying process. (Thin-skinned legumes like lentils or split peas do not require soaking.) There are two methods of soaking. For the longer method, which eliminates up to 90 percent of the indigestible sugars that produce gas and bloating, simply immerse the legumes in boiling water and let them soak for at least eight hours in the refrigerator. Be sure to discard the soaking water and add fresh water for cooking. To quick-soak, place the legumes in a pot, add hot water to cover, bring to a boil for two minutes, cover and then let stand for one hour. Again, discard the soaking water before cooking.

To cook dried beans, use three cups of water per cup of beans. Bring the water slowly to a boil and skim off the starchy scum that rises to the surface. It is very important that dried legumes be boiled long enough to destroy their lectins, toxins that can cause gastrointes-

PREPARING LEGUMES

Many of the recipes in this volume call for cooked legumes. Except for split peas and lentils, the legumes listed below should be soaked before cooking. Procedures for soaking and cooking are explained at right. Remember that most legumes will more than double in volume during cooking.

BLACK BEANS *Boil, uncovered, for 10 minutes, using 3 parts water to 1 part beans, then simmer, covered, 1 to 1 1/2 hours.*

CHICKPEAS *Boil, uncovered, for 10 minutes, using 3 parts water to 1 part chickpeas, then simmer, covered, 2 1/2 to 3 hours.*

KIDNEY BEANS, NAVY BEANS, PINTO BEANS, WHITE BEANS *Boil, uncovered, for 10 minutes, using 3 parts water to 1 part beans, then simmer, covered, for 1 1/2 to 2 hours.*

LENTILS *Boil, uncovered, for 2 minutes, using 3 parts water to 1 part lentils, then simmer, covered, for 20 to 25 minutes.*

SPLIT PEAS *Boil, uncovered, for 2 minutes, using 4 parts water to 1 part peas, then simmer, covered, for 30 minutes.*

Buying and Storing Guide

◆ When purchasing legumes in bulk, look for consistency in size and color. Beans should be bright in color — age fades them — and free of dirt, debris and mold. Avoid cracked beans or any with pinhole marks, possible signs of insect damage. Shop for beans in stores that have a high turnover of merchandise. Bins of loose beans should be cleaned and restocked frequently.

◆ Dried peas and beans should be uniform in size so that they will cook at the same rate. Do not mix newly bought dried legumes with old ones, since they will cook unevenly. Older beans take longer to cook. Fresh beans such as lima beans should look plump and unshriveled.

◆ Uncooked legumes can be stored in a sealed package or a tightly closed container for up to a year in a cool, dry place. Cooked beans will last three to four days in a covered container in the refrigerator, and between four and six months in the freezer.

◆ Canned legumes usually cost more and take up more space than the dried varieties, but they have the same shelf life and are the quickest to prepare, since they only require reheating. However, the texture of canned beans often suffers in processing, which can make them mushy.

tinal distress. Most dried legumes should be boiled for at least 10 minutes to destroy these lectins; lentils and split peas need to be boiled for just two or three minutes. If you are concerned about flatulence, discard the boiling water, too. Otherwise, you can use it as stock for making soup.

After boiling, bring the water to a simmer and continue to cook the legumes. Cooking times — including boiling — range from less than an hour for lentils to two and a half to three hours for chickpeas. In general, cook legumes, stirring occasionally and adding water as necessary, until they are tender but not mushy. Legumes will more than double in volume during cooking. A pound of dried beans (just over two cups) generally cooks up to about four cups.

Legumes readily take on the flavor of whatever they are cooked with, such as herbs, spices or vegetables. Acidic ingredients such as tomatoes, wine, lemon juice or vinegar should be added only toward the end of cooking, since the acid slows the softening process and thus extends the cooking time.

Many legumes can also be purchased precooked in cans or frozen — a time-saver if you are in a rush. While canned peas and beans retain most of their original nutrients, they are often high in sodium. Be sure to drain and rinse them thoroughly before using in order to remove some of this excess sodium.

As the following recipes demonstrate, you can use legumes in a variety of interesting and healthful dishes — from soups and salads to main courses. Feel free to experiment. Mixing different kinds of legumes can often make a recipe more interesting.

CHICKPEA AND ESCAROLE SOUP

CALORIES	183
61% Carbohydrate	29 g
15% Protein	7 g
24% Fat	5 g
CALCIUM	81 mg
IRON	3 mg
SODIUM	468 mg

The combination of rice and chickpeas in this recipe provides as complete a protein as you would get in meat but with much less fat and no cholesterol.

2 tablespoons olive oil
1 cup chopped onion
1 tablespoon minced garlic
1 1/2 teaspoons minced fresh thyme, or 1/2 teaspoon dried thyme, crumbled
1 1/2 teaspoons minced fresh oregano, or 1/2 teaspoon dried oregano, crushed
1/4 cup long-grain white rice

2 1/2 cups cooked chickpeas (1 1/4 cups dried)
8 cups coarsely chopped escarole leaves
1 cup frozen or canned corn kernels
2 tablespoons tomato paste
2 tablespoons lemon juice
1 1/2 teaspoons salt
1/4 teaspoon hot pepper sauce
Black pepper

In a 6- to 8-quart pot, heat the oil over medium heat. Stir in the onion, garlic, thyme and oregano and sauté 3 to 5 minutes, or until the onion is wilted. Add the rice, chickpeas and escarole, and stir to coat lightly with oil. Add 10 cups of water, cover the pot and bring to a boil. Reduce the heat and simmer, covered, 30 minutes. Stir in the corn, tomato paste and lemon juice. Return the soup to a boil, cover and simmer 30 minutes. Add the salt and hot pepper sauce, and pepper to taste, and serve. Makes 8 servings

Note: This soup freezes well. Freeze it in single servings for quick meals.

WHITE BEAN AND CORN SOUP

CALORIES	305
66% Carbohydrate	52 g
18% Protein	14 g
16% Fat	6 g
CALCIUM	187 mg
IRON	4 mg
SODIUM	391 mg

Dried beans are lower in sodium than canned ones. If you cook with canned beans, you can eliminate much of the added salt by rinsing and draining the beans before using them.

2 strips bacon, diced
1/2 cup diced onion
2 garlic cloves, minced
1/2 cup coarsely chopped carrot
3/4 cup coarsely diced red bell pepper
1 1/2 tablespoons unbleached all-purpose flour

1 cup skim milk
1 bay leaf
1/2 teaspoon salt
1/4 teaspoon white pepper
1/4 teaspoon sage
1 1/2 cups cooked white beans (3/4 cup dried)
1 cup frozen or canned corn kernels

In a medium-size saucepan over medium-low heat, cook the bacon about 6 minutes, or until crisp; pour off all but 1 tablespoon of fat. Add the onion, garlic, carrot and bell pepper to the saucepan and cook, covered, about 7 minutes, or until the vegetables are softened. Add the flour and cook, stirring, 1 minute. Add 1 cup of water, the milk, bay leaf, salt, pepper and sage, and cook another 4 minutes, or until the soup is slightly thickened. Add the beans and cook another 10 minutes, or until the flavors are well blended. Add the corn and cook just until heated through. Makes 4 servings

Chickpea and Escarole Soup ▷

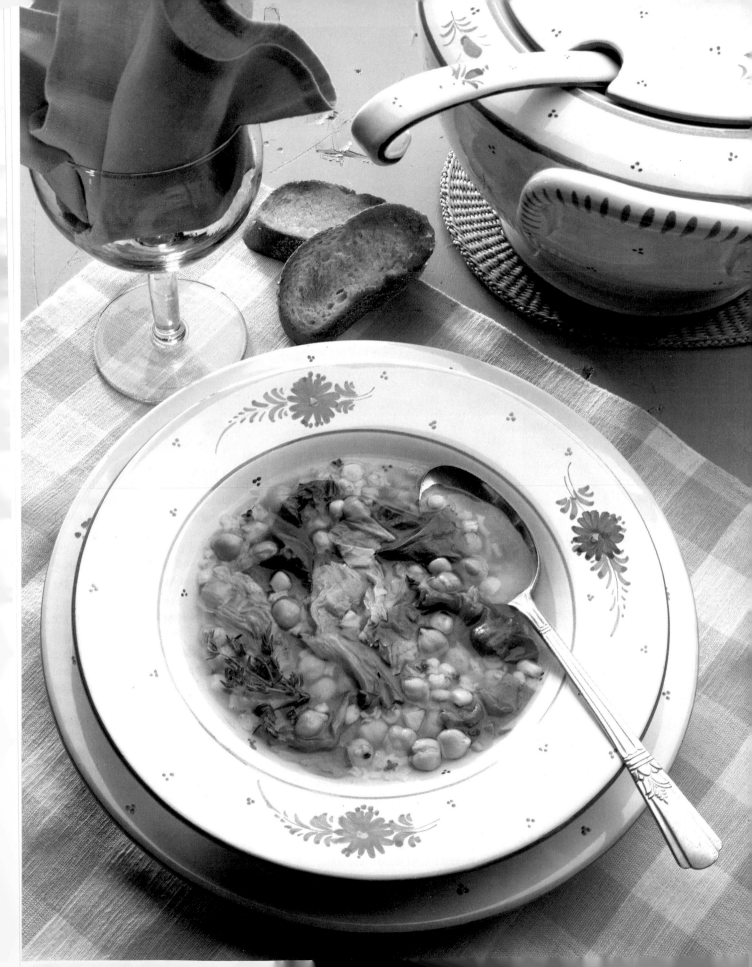

LENTIL CROQUETTES WITH SPICY RAITA

CALORIES without Raita	323
58% Carbohydrate	48 g
19% Protein	16 g
23% Fat	8 g
CALCIUM	79 mg
IRON	4 mg
SODIUM	497 mg

A half cup of lentils provides 15 percent of your daily requirement of copper, a mineral that is necessary for making red blood cells and important for absorbing and using iron. This recipe also supplies more than 20 percent of your daily iron requirement.

2 1/4 cups cooked lentils, cooked very soft (1 cup dried)
1 cup minced onion
1 teaspoon minced garlic
1/2 teaspoon salt
1/4 teaspoon ground cumin

1/4 teaspoon curry powder
1/8 teaspoon celery salt
3/4 cup dry bread crumbs
2 tablespoons vegetable oil
Spicy Raita (recipe follows)

Preheat the oven to 350° F. In a medium-size bowl, stir together the lentils, onion, garlic, salt and spices. Stir in half of the bread crumbs. With wet hands, shape the lentil mixture into 8 patties. Spread the remaining bread crumbs on a plate. One at a time, dredge the patties in the crumbs, turning to coat them

Lentil Croquettes with Spicy Raita

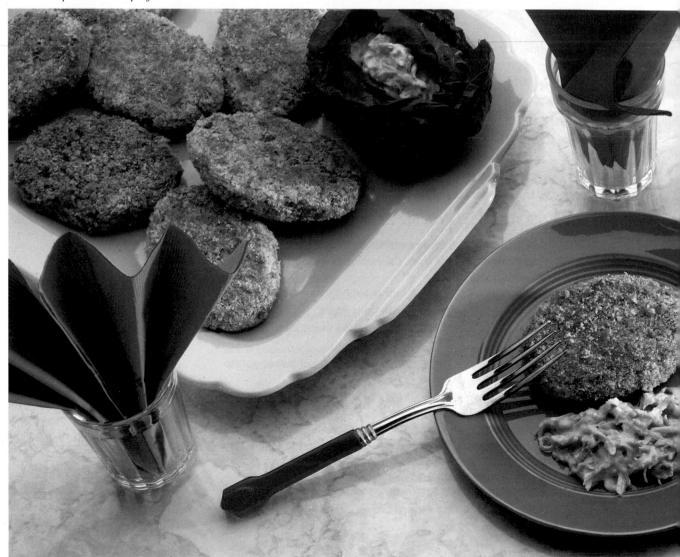

evenly. Heat the oil in a large ovenproof skillet over medium-low heat until the surface ripples. Fry the croquettes 2 minutes on each side, or until crisp and browned, then place the skillet in the oven and bake 20 minutes. Serve the croquettes with Spicy Raita.   Makes 4 servings

SPICY RAITA

Raita, an Indian condiment, is a combination of yogurt, spices and chopped vegetables or fruit.

1 cup grated carrot
1/2 cup plain lowfat yogurt
1/2 cup thinly sliced scallion
1 tablespoon honey

1 1/2 teaspoons olive oil
1/2 teaspoon minced garlic
1/2 teaspoon red pepper flakes
Black pepper to taste

CALORIES	65
59% Carbohydrate	10 g
12% Protein	2 g
29% Fat	2 g
CALCIUM	68 mg
IRON	.4 mg
SODIUM	30 mg

Combine all the ingredients in a small bowl and stir together until smooth. Refrigerate the raita until ready to serve.   Makes 4 servings

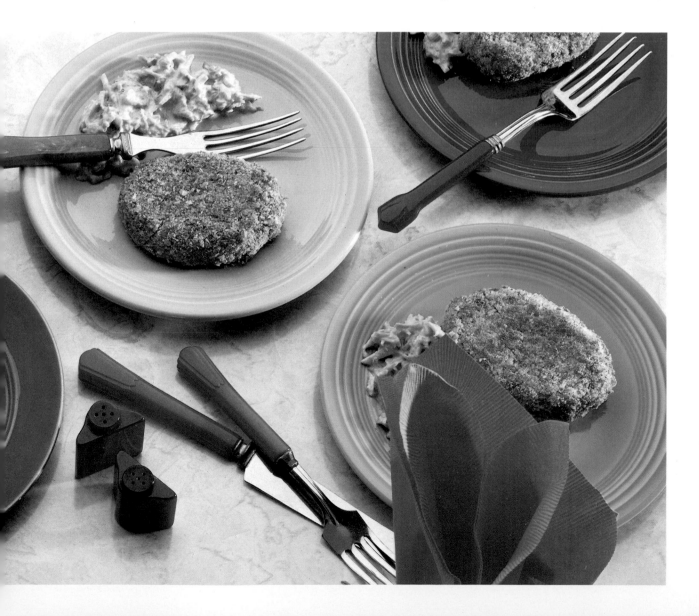

SPLIT PEA STEW WITH SPICY MEATBALLS

CALORIES	399
57% Carbohydrate	59 g
17% Protein	17 g
26% Fat	12 g
CALCIUM	64 mg
IRON	3 mg
SODIUM	457 mg

While ground beef alone provides complete protein, it is high in fat and cholesterol. This hearty stew recipe uses less meat than a typical beef or lamb stew, but it includes lots of satisfying winter vegetables, and split peas as a complementary high-fiber protein source.

1/4 pound ground beef
1 cup chopped onion
1/4 cup dry bread crumbs
1/2 teaspoon red pepper flakes, crushed
1/4 teaspoon fennel seeds, crushed
1/4 teaspoon dried rosemary, crushed
1/4 teaspoon celery salt

2 tablespoons olive oil
1 cup grated carrot
2 cups cooked yellow split peas (1 cup dried)
2 cups diced cooked parsnips
1 1/2 cups peeled, diced, boiled potatoes
1 tablespoon honey
1/2 teaspoon salt
Black pepper

Preheat the oven to 350° F. In a medium-size bowl, gently toss together the ground beef, 1/4 cup of the onion, the bread crumbs, red pepper flakes, fennel seeds, rosemary and celery salt. Handle the mixture lightly; overworking will toughen the meat. Stir in 2 tablespoons of water. Shape the mixture into 8 meatballs, place them in a baking dish and bake about 15 minutes, or until browned. Set aside.

In a large saucepan, heat the oil over medium heat. Stir in the remaining onion and the carrots and sauté 3 to 5 minutes, or until the vegetables are wilted. Add the peas, parsnips, potatoes, honey, salt, pepper to taste and 2 cups of water, and stir. Add the meatballs, increase the heat to medium-high and bring the stew to a boil. Reduce the heat to medium-low, cover and simmer 20 to 30 minutes, or until the stew is slightly thickened.

Makes 4 servings

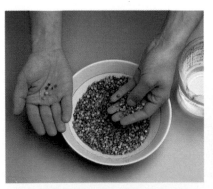

After removing any discolored peas and debris, place the peas in a bowl, cover with cold water and, after a minute or so, remove any peas that float to the surface.

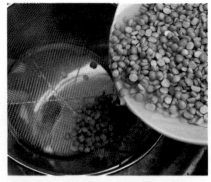

Drain the peas into a colander and rinse under cold running water. While most dried legumes need soaking to rehydrate them before cooking, split peas do not.

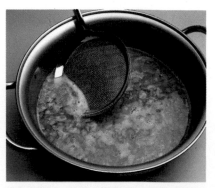

Bring the peas to a boil over medium heat. Using a skimmer or large spoon, remove the scum that rises to the surface. Repeat as necessary as the peas cook.

CHICKPEA AND LIMA BEAN CASSEROLE

A half cup of chickpeas contains more than 40 percent of your daily requirement of folacin, a B vitamin necessary for red-blood-cell production.

CALORIES	188
71% Carbohydrate	34 g
21% Protein	10 g
8% Fat	2 g
CALCIUM	87 mg
IRON	3 mg
SODIUM	229 mg

2 cups cooked chickpeas (1 cup dried)
One 10-ounce package frozen lima beans, thawed
One 3/4-pound eggplant, cut into 1/4-inch dice (3 1/2 cups)
1/4 cup plus 3 tablespoons low-sodium chicken stock
1/2 cup chopped onion
2 garlic cloves, minced
2 tablespoons minced fresh ginger
1 tablespoon unbleached all-purpose flour
3 small fresh plum tomatoes, peeled, seeded and chopped
1 teaspoon ground cumin
1/2 teaspoon salt
1/8 teaspoon Cayenne pepper
2 tablespoons chopped fresh coriander

Preheat the oven to 350° F. In a 2-quart casserole, combine the chickpeas, lima beans, eggplant and 1 cup of water; set aside. In a medium-size skillet heat 3 tablespoons of stock over medium heat. Add the onion and garlic, and cook 2 minutes. Add the ginger and cook another 2 minutes. Add the flour and cook, stirring, 1 minute. Add the remaining stock, the tomatoes, cumin, salt and Cayenne, and cook, stirring, another minute. Pour the mixture into the casserole, stir, cover with foil and bake 1 hour. Sprinkle the casserole with coriander and serve.   Makes 6 servings

KIDNEY BEAN AND TUNA SALAD

Kidney beans, like other dried beans, are among the least processed foods in the supermarket. They are usually not heated intensely or treated with preservatives, as many other foods are.

1 1/2 cups cooked kidney beans (1/2 cup dried)
One 6 1/2-ounce can water-packed tuna, drained and flaked
1/2 cup diced red bell pepper
1/2 cup chopped fresh Italian parsley
2 tablespoons chopped fresh coriander
1/2 cup diced celery
1/4 cup lemon juice
3 tablespoons low-sodium chicken stock
2 1/2 teaspoons minced garlic
1/4 teaspoon hot pepper sauce
1/8 teaspoon salt
1/8 teaspoon black pepper

CALORIES	104
52% Carbohydrate	14 g
43% Protein	11 g
5% Fat	1 g
CALCIUM	39 mg
IRON	2 mg
SODIUM	174 mg

Place the beans in a large bowl. Add the tuna, bell pepper, parsley, coriander and celery, and toss well. For the dressing, whisk together the lemon juice, stock, garlic, hot pepper sauce, salt and pepper in a small bowl. Pour the dressing over the bean mixture and toss gently to combine. Set aside at room temperature for 1 hour to allow the flavors to blend.   Makes 6 servings

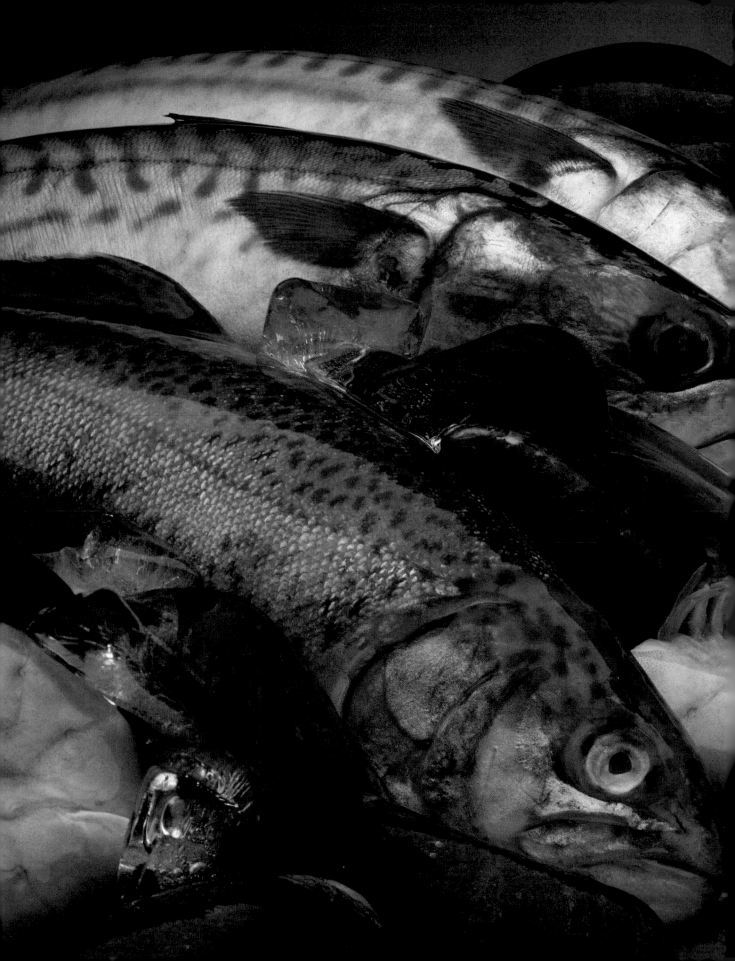

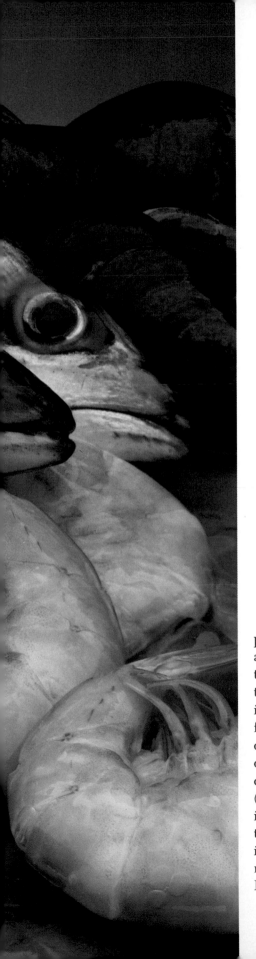

CHAPTER SIX

Seafood

*Rich in protein and minerals
with a healthy kind of fat*

Seafood excels as a source of protein — most varieties contain at least 75 percent protein — as well as of minerals and B vitamins. Most fish are also relatively low in fat, though some varieties do contain nearly as much fat as lean meat. But the fat in fish, which takes the form of oil, is highly polyunsaturated, so it is preferable to the fat in meat, which is largely saturated. In fact, fish oil contains a unique group of polyunsaturated fatty acids, called omega-3 acids, which appear to offer double benefits: They not only decrease levels of artery-choking LDL (low-density lipoprotein) cholesterol, but also may raise levels of the artery-clearing HDL (high-density lipoprotein) cholesterol. One study found a reassuring inverse relationship between fish consumption and heart disease — the more fish consumed by the general population, the lower the incidence of heart disease. Further research indicates that this benefit may be independent of such factors as weight, stress and exercise. Fish oil also helps prevent hardening of the arteries by thinning the

93

blood, thereby making it less likely to stick to the walls of blood vessels, and by reducing the likelihood of arterial blood clots. Finally, fish oil is rich in vitamins A and D.

Researchers have found that the higher the fat content of seafood, the greater the cardiovascular benefits, and the darker the flesh of a fish, the more oil it contains. Fatty fish — those that contain from five to 20 percent fat — include deepwater fish like tuna and swordfish (their fat-marbled flesh helps to insulate them against cold water), as well as anchovies, herring, mackerel, salmon and sardines. Fish that have between two and five percent fat include bass, bluefish, halibut, ocean perch, pollock, rockfish and smelt. Lean fish contain less than two percent fat and include flatfish like flounder and sole.

Although shellfish were once considered high in cholesterol, new methods of food analysis have revealed that most shellfish contain less cholesterol than the moderate amounts found in other fish. Lobster has only slightly more cholesterol than beef or chicken. Mussels, clams and oysters, which are low in cholesterol, have now been shown to be proportionately high in omega-3 fatty acids.

Seafood, especially shellfish, is very rich in minerals — most notably iron and fluorine. Ocean fish are the best natural source of iodine, which is important in the production of hormones in the thyroid gland. Seafood also supplies some B vitamins, including thiamin, riboflavin and niacin. (Fish roe, or fish eggs, are especially rich in thiamin and riboflavin.) The edible bones of canned salmon and sardines are excellent sources of calcium.

Because of its many benefits, nutritionists recommend eating seafood, lean or fatty, at least once a week, and the immense variety of fish and shellfish available at fish markets and supermarkets should make this easy. Because fresh seafood is quite perishable, its regional availability is often limited. If you cannot find the specific type of fish that a recipe calls for, substitute a species that is similar in taste and texture. Cook fresh fish within two days of buying it. While using frozen fish is acceptable, the freezing process makes the fish tougher.

The type, cut and fattiness of a fish determine which cooking method is most suitable. Flatfish are usually cooked whole or cut into fillets. They can then be broiled, sautéed, baked, steamed or poached. Because flatfish tend to be dry, fat often needs to be added when cooking them. You should use unsaturated vegetable oil.

Fatty fish can be cooked whole, divided into fillets or cut crosswise into steaks. While these fish can be cooked by any of the methods used for flatfish, it is best not to sauté them, since their flesh is sufficiently rich without adding butter or cooking oil.

Shellfish such as clams, mussels, oysters, scallops and small shrimp should be steamed, boiled, broiled or sautéed. Larger, moister shellfish like jumbo shrimp and lobster can also be baked. It is important to note that eating raw shellfish, even if it is certified as clean, can be dangerous because of bacterial or viral contamination from polluted waters. Similarly, inadequately cooked shellfish can be harmful to

Buying and Storing Guide

◆ Always check fish for freshness before purchasing it. Whole fish should have firm flesh that springs back when touched, as well as tight scales, red gills and bright, bulging eyes. Fillets and steaks should be moist and transparent. Fish should smell fresh — not fishy.

◆ When buying whole fish, allow one pound per person; dressed fish (cleaned, with head and tail removed), 3/4 pound per person; and steaks and fillets, 1/3 to 1/2 pound per person. Store fish in the coldest part of the refrigerator, loosely covered with plastic wrap.

◆ When shopping for frozen fish, make sure that it is completely covered in moisture-proof wrap. The flesh should be solid, with no odor. Avoid misshapen or torn packages and packages that contain blood. You can keep fatty frozen fish at 0° F for three months; leaner frozen fish keeps for up to six months.

◆ Shellfish can sometimes be contaminated by toxic bacteria and viruses. Harvesting is state-monitored, but you should still buy shellfish from such reliable sources as supermarkets and established fish stores. Store shellfish below 40° F and use it quickly.

your health. For instance, steaming clams for only one minute does not heat them sufficiently to kill any viruses they may harbor. All the recipes in this book give safe cooking times for shellfish.

For the best taste and texture, along with the most nutrients, do not overcook seafood. Fish cooks quickly because it has little connective tissue; moderate cooking temperatures are best. The fish is done if it is opaque, does not cling to the bones and flakes easily when pierced at its thickest point with a fork. A good rule for cooking whole fish, fillets and steaks is to allow 10 minutes for each inch of thickness, measured at the thickest point (although thin fillets cook more quickly and should be watched carefully). Double this time for frozen fish. Shellfish like shrimp and scallops are done when they are no longer translucent. Shellfish like clams and mussels are done when their shells open.

Canned fish can also be used inventively in many recipes. When possible, buy fish that has been packed in water; fish packed in oil has twice the calories. If you must use oil-packed fish, drain the oil and rinse the fish under running water to reduce the excess calories. Rinsing canned fish, whether packed in water or oil, will also remove almost all the extra sodium that is added during canning: Processing generally adds four to 10 times the amount of sodium that is found in fresh varieties.

Seafood should not be limited to main courses. Consider using it in appetizers, salads and side dishes, starting with some of the following recipes. And remember that combining seafood with vegetables and pasta enhances its versatility.

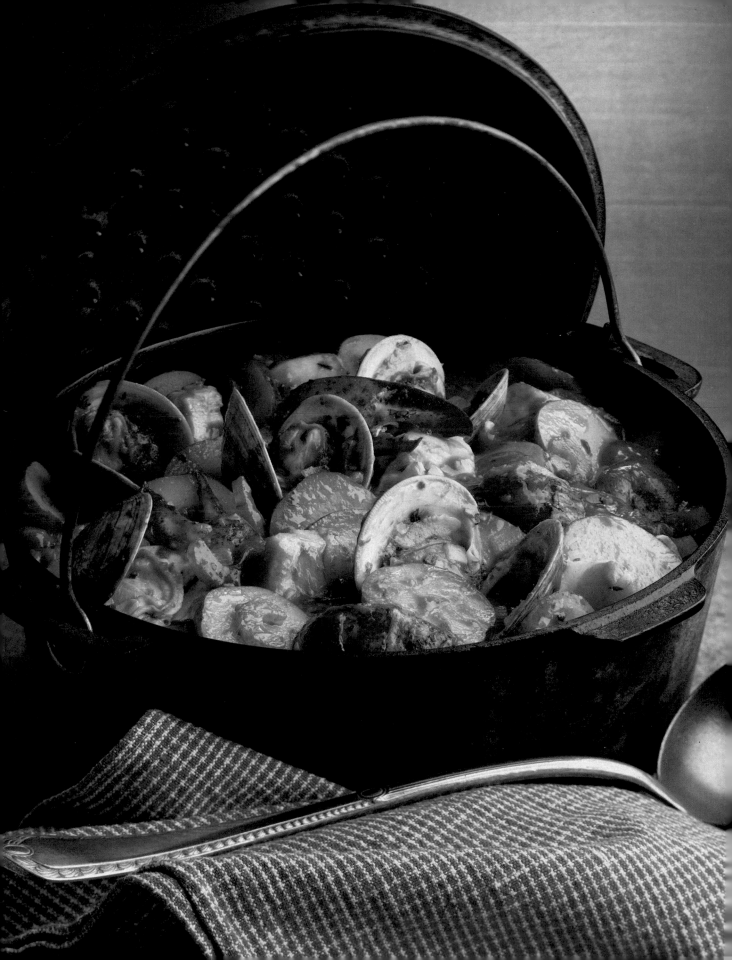

SEAFOOD STEW

Although many people believe that lobster is loaded with cholesterol, 3 1/2 ounces of lobster meat has less cholesterol than one egg. And lobster is rich in potassium, which helps maintain the body's proper fluid balance.

CALORIES	306
44% Carbohydrate	34 g
37% Protein	28 g
19% Fat	6 g
CALCIUM	149 mg
IRON	7 mg
SODIUM	496 mg

2 tablespoons olive oil
2 garlic cloves, minced
1 cup chopped onion
1 cup chopped celery
1 1/4 pounds potatoes, cut into 1/4-inch-thick slices
1 teaspoon saffron threads, or less to taste
2 tablespoons chopped fresh basil, or 2 teaspoons dried basil
1 teaspoon dried thyme
1/2 teaspoon red pepper flakes
1 cup dry vermouth
One 35-ounce can Italian plum tomatoes
One 1 1/4-pound lobster, cut into 1 1/2-inch chunks
12 cherrystone clams, scrubbed
1 pound cod, cut into 1 1/2-inch chunks

Heat the oil in a large pot over medium heat. Add the garlic and onion and cook about 5 minutes, or until the onion is soft. Add the celery, potatoes, saffron, basil, thyme, red pepper flakes, vermouth and tomatoes with their liquid; stir well. Bring the stew to a boil, then reduce the heat and simmer, covered, 15 minutes. Add the lobster and clams and cook another 10 minutes. Add the cod and cook 10 minutes longer.   Makes 6 servings

Note: You can use other types of fresh fish and seafood in this recipe. For instance, try substituting halibut, mussels or any type of small clams if the suggested ingredients are not available.

Despite the popularity of high-protein weight-loss diets, there is no evidence that eating a lot of protein-rich foods contributes to long-term weight reduction. No matter what kinds of foods you eat, if you take in more calories than you use, those incoming calories will be stored in your body as fat.

PASTA WITH SPINACH AND CLAMS

Like all shellfish, the clams in this recipe are rich in iodine, which is necessary for the regulation of energy release within muscle cells.

1 cup finely chopped onion
2 garlic cloves, minced
1/2 cup white wine or dry vermouth
6 ounces medium-size shell pasta
2 dozen shucked clams, coarsely chopped, liquid reserved
2 cups blanched, coarsely chopped spinach
1/4 cup low-sodium chicken stock
2 tablespoons lemon juice
2 teaspoons olive oil, preferably extra-virgin
1/4 teaspoon grated lemon peel
1/4 teaspoon salt
1/8 teaspoon red pepper flakes

Bring a large pot of water to a boil. In a medium-size nonstick skillet, cook the onions and garlic in the wine over medium heat, covered, for about 10 minutes, or until soft. Meanwhile, cook the pasta in the boiling water according to the package directions until al dente; drain and return the pasta to the pot to keep warm. Reserving the liquid, add the clams to the skillet and cook, stirring, about 3 minutes, or until the clams are tender. Pour the contents of the skillet over the pasta and toss gently. Add the reserved clam liquid and the remaining ingredients, mix well and serve.   Makes 4 servings

CALORIES	276
64% Carbohydrate	43 g
24% Protein	16 g
12% Fat	4 g
CALCIUM	122 mg
IRON	9 mg
SODIUM	343 mg

◁ *Seafood Stew*

PROVENÇAL SEAFOOD PIZZA

A typical cheese-laden pizza derives most of its calories from fat. This seafood-topped pie is lower in fat and higher in carbohydrates.

Crust:
1 package fast-rising yeast
Pinch of sugar
2/3 cup warm water (115° F)
1 3/4 cups unbleached all-purpose flour
1/2 teaspoon salt
1 teaspoon olive oil

Topping:
2 tablespoons olive oil
8 cups sliced onions (2 pounds)

1 cup low-sodium tomato sauce
1 garlic clove, minced
1/4 teaspoon salt
Pinch of dried thyme
1/4 pound medium-size shelled, deveined shrimp, tails left intact if desired
1/4 pound bay scallops
3 anchovy fillets, halved
6 small black olives

For the crust, in a small bowl dissolve the yeast and sugar in the water. Place the flour, salt and oil in a food processor. Start the machine, add the yeast

CALORIES	218
59% Carbohydrate	32 g
19% Protein	10 g
22% Fat	5 g
CALCIUM	48 mg
IRON	2 mg
SODIUM	284 mg

mixture and process 45 seconds. Transfer the dough to a large plastic bag and set aside to rise 25 minutes.

Meanwhile, for the topping, heat 1 1/2 tablespoons of oil in a nonstick skillet over medium-low heat. Add the onions and cook, covered, 25 to 30 minutes, stirring occasionally. Watch the onions closely during the last 10 minutes and, when golden and dry, remove them from the skillet to cool.

While the onions are cooking, make the sauce. Combine the tomato sauce, garlic, salt and thyme in a small saucepan, bring to a boil and simmer 8 minutes, or until the sauce is slightly thickened; transfer the sauce to a measuring cup or small pitcher and set aside.

Roll out the crust to fit a 12-inch pizza pan, place it in the pan and let it rise in a warm place 10 minutes. Meanwhile, heat the remaining 1/2 tablespoon of oil in the skillet over medium-high heat and sauté the shrimp and scallops 1 minute, or until opaque. Remove the skillet from the heat and set aside.

Preheat the oven to 425° F. Spread the onions evenly over the crust. Pour the tomato sauce over the onions. Arrange the seafood on top of the sauce and garnish the pizza with anchovies and olives. Bake the pizza 20 minutes, or until the crust is golden. Let the pizza cool 5 minutes, then cut into 8 wedges and serve.   Makes 8 servings

SEAFOOD RAREBIT

This dish eliminates most of the saturated fat usually present in rarebit by cutting back on the amount of cheese. But it still supplies a fair amount of calcium — more than 15 percent of your daily need per serving.

CALORIES	337
45% Carbohydrate	38 g
26% Protein	22 g
29% Fat	11 g
CALCIUM	210 mg
IRON	3 mg
SODIUM	805 mg

1/4 pound monkfish or other white-fleshed fish fillets
1/2 cup frozen or canned crabmeat, drained, liquid reserved
1 teaspoon olive oil
2 teaspoons minced shallots
1/2 cup white wine
1/2 red bell pepper, roasted and peeled (see page 40)
3/4 cup shredded extra-sharp Cheddar cheese
1/4 cup unbleached all-purpose flour
1 teaspoon Dijon-style mustard
1/4 teaspoon salt
1/4 cup lowfat milk
4 English muffins
16 fresh or frozen asparagus spears, blanched

Cut the fish into 1 × 3/8-inch pieces. Place the reserved liquid from the crabmeat in a measuring cup and add enough water to measure 1 cup; set aside. Heat the oil in a medium-size saucepan over medium-low heat. Add the shallots and sauté 4 minutes. Add the crab liquid and wine and bring to a simmer. Add the fish and cook about 2 minutes, or until opaque. Remove the pan from the heat. Reserving the cooking liquid, remove the fish; set aside.

Preheat the broiler. Dice the bell pepper. Combine 1/2 cup of the reserved cooking liquid, half of the bell pepper, the cheese, flour, mustard and salt in a food processor or blender. Process about 2 minutes, or until blended. Add the cheese mixture and milk to the cooking liquid remaining in the saucepan, increase the heat to medium and bring to a boil. Reduce the heat and simmer 4 minutes, stirring occasionally. Add the remaining bell pepper, the crabmeat and fish, and cook another 2 minutes, or until heated through. Meanwhile, split the muffins and toast until lightly browned. Place 2 asparagus spears on each muffin half, top each with 1/2 cup of the rarebit mixture and broil 5 inches from the heat about 4 minutes, or until bubbly.   Makes 4 servings

MUSSELS WITH TOMATO COULIS

Like all shellfish, mussels are rich in iron.

8 mussels, well scrubbed
2 tablespoons dry vermouth
1 teaspoon olive oil
1 large garlic clove, minced
1/2 cup chopped onion
1 pound fresh plum tomatoes, coarsely chopped
1/2 teaspoon dried oregano, crushed

CALORIES	68
48% Carbohydrate	9 g
26% Protein	5 g
26% Fat	2 g
CALCIUM	26 mg
IRON	2 mg
SODIUM	91 mg

Place the mussels and vermouth in a small saucepan, cover and cook over medium-high heat about 5 minutes, or until the mussels open; discard any that do not open. Strain and reserve the liquid. Shell the mussels; set aside. For the coulis, heat the oil in a large skillet over medium-high heat. Add the garlic and onion and cook 2 minutes, or until soft. Add the mussel liquid, tomatoes and oregano and cook over high heat 10 minutes, or until thick; transfer to a bowl and let cool to room temperature. Divide the coulis among 4 salad plates and arrange the mussels on top.   Makes 4 servings

PASTA PRIMAVERA SALAD WITH SALMON

The salmon and asparagus in this recipe supply more than 25 percent of your daily vitamin A requirement.

1/2 pound rotelle or other spiral pasta

2 pounds asparagus, trimmed and cut into 2-inch pieces

1 1/2 cups julienned cucumber

1 cup julienned zucchini

One 10-ounce package frozen peas, thawed

1/4 cup lemon juice

1 tablespoon grated lemon peel

1 tablespoon olive oil, preferably extra-virgin

1/4 pound salmon fillet, poached and flaked

1/4 teaspoon salt

1/4 teaspoon pepper

CALORIES	217
57% Carbohydrate	32 g
24% Protein	13 g
19% Fat	5 g
CALCIUM	62 mg
IRON	2 mg
SODIUM	126 mg

Bring 2 large pots of water to a boil. In one pot, cook the pasta according to the package directions until al dente; drain, rinse, drain again and set aside in a large bowl. In the other pot of boiling water, blanch the asparagus about 3 minutes, or until crisp-tender; drain, cool slightly and add to the pasta. Add the cucumber, zucchini, peas, lemon juice, peel and oil, and toss to combine. Add the salmon, salt and pepper, and toss gently.   Makes 8 servings

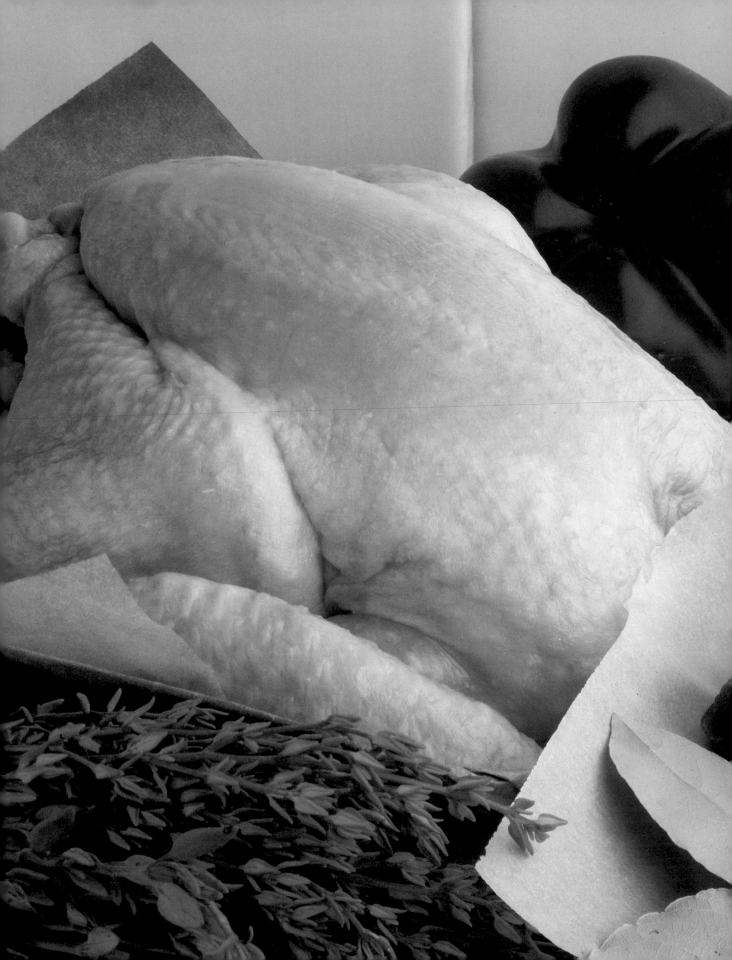

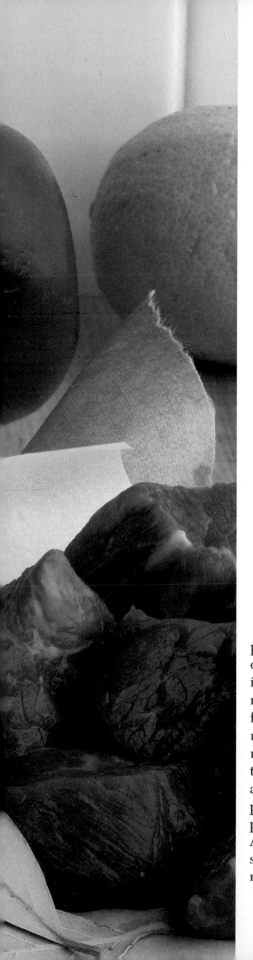

CHAPTER SEVEN

Meat and Poultry

Quality, not quantity

More than two thirds of the protein in the American diet comes from animals, particularly beef cattle. While the protein in meat and poultry is of good quality — that is, it contains a complete complement of essential amino acids — this nutritional value is often overshadowed by the high levels of saturated fat and cholesterol in many meats. Fortunately, meat producers have reduced the fat content of their products: According to a U.S. Department of Agriculture study, cattle are approximately 25 percent leaner than they were 30 years ago, and pork is a full 50 percent leaner. Since a single three-ounce serving of cooked lean meat or poultry supplies 40 to 55 percent of the Recommended Dietary Allowance of protein for an adult male, and 50 to 60 percent for a woman, most Americans need not worry about getting enough protein. Instead, they should be learning how to prepare meals using smaller amounts of meat and poultry.

Meat is also one of the best food sources of iron. One three-ounce serving of beef or lamb provides virtually all the Recommended Dietary Allowance of iron for a man, and about 50 percent for a woman. The iron in meat is in a form called heme iron, which is three to five times more easily absorbed by the body than the iron in other foods. And, when meat is consumed with less readily absorbed iron in such foods as spinach, an unidentified substance in the meat acts as a catalyst for iron absorption.

In addition, meat supplies a good amount of other minerals, in particular zinc, phosphorus, potassium and copper. All meats contribute B vitamins (niacin, riboflavin and thiamin) to the diet. In fact, fresh pork is by far the best source of thiamin — it contains more than twice as much per serving as any other food. Vitamin A, iron, copper, riboflavin and niacin are most concentrated in the liver of animals. But liver and other organ meats are also quite high in cholesterol, so you should eat them no more than once a week.

The main concern about meat in your diet should be to limit the amount of *fatty* meat you eat. Untrimmed fatty meat often contains 50 percent more calories than well-trimmed lean beef, and up to 70 percent of those calories come from fat (compared with 30 to 45 percent in lean beef). Ironically, the most expensive cuts of meat are often the highest in fat, due to the amount of marbling (the flecks of fat scattered throughout) required for tenderness. Leaner cuts of meat come from the animal's most-used muscles, such as the shoulder, flank and neck. These cuts are generally less expensive because they are less tender, but you can tenderize them with proper cooking. Ground beef, which accounts for almost 40 percent of all beef consumed in the United States, can be purchased in lowfat grades. Veal is another good lowfat meat, although it is somewhat higher in cholesterol than other meats.

Another solution to the fatty-meat dilemma is to eat more chicken and turkey, which contain considerably less fat than red meat. Removing the skin from poultry cuts its fat content in half. Skinless chicken or turkey breast, for example, has more protein than fatty steak, but only about one tenth the fat and half the calories. Purchase smaller, younger birds, which are less fatty than older birds. Goose and duck are high in fat, so you should eat them infrequently.

Poultry has many of the same nutritional benefits as meat. In fact, chicken and turkey breasts have even more niacin than lean meat, with younger chickens having the most. Dark-meat poultry is rich in riboflavin and thiamin. Unfortunately, the cholesterol levels in poultry are also comparable to those of meat — between 60 and 70 milligrams in a three-ounce serving, or about one fifth the maximum daily intake recommended by the American Heart Association. Little of this cholesterol is in the fat. So although removing fatty skin or trimming off fat cuts calories, reducing cholesterol intake requires eating smaller portions.

Properly prepared, lean meat and poultry are tender, flavorful and nutritious. Before cooking meat, trim all visible fat. You can cook meat

Buying and Storing Guide

Purchase the leanest grades of meat possible. The U.S. Department of Agriculture grades meat by color and marbling, which indicate tenderness, juiciness and flavor. Consumers can choose from three grades of beef, Prime, Choice and Good; the Good grade has less marbling and surrounding fat than the higher-priced Prime and Choice grades. Store-branded "lean" beef is most likely Good grade. Veal comes in only Prime and Choice, but its fat content is lower than that of beef.

The cut of meat determines its fat content. Top round, shoulder, flank, eye round, top sirloin and extra-lean ground are among the leanest types of beef. There is less variation in the fat content of different cuts of pork, lamb and veal than of beef.

The best beef is bright red with firm, ivory-colored fat; the best veal is light pinkish-white, also with ivory-colored fat. Fresh pork should be firm-textured and grayish-pink to deep rose in color, with some marbling and a layer of white exterior fat. Trim all visible fat from meat before cooking it.

Store fresh meat in the coldest part of your refrigerator. Large cuts of meat (steaks or roasts) can be refrigerated for three to four days, smaller cuts for two to three days and ground meat for one or two days. Freeze large cuts of meat for no more than nine months, ground meat for up to three months.

Chicken is classified as a roaster, broiler, fryer or stewing hen. Small roasters are the lowest in fat and the tenderest; stewing hens are the least tender and are often used in soups. Chicken will keep in the coldest part of your refrigerator for one or two days and can be frozen for up to 12 months. Turkey can be refrigerated for up to a week and frozen for six months. Thaw frozen poultry in the refrigerator.

using dry-heat methods, such as roasting, baking and broiling, or by moist-heat methods, such as poaching, braising and steaming. Broiling and roasting allow excess fat to drip away, while moist-heat methods tenderize leaner cuts. As a general rule, meat from younger animals cooks more quickly than meat from older animals. If fat is needed for basting purposes, brush the meat with a little vegetable oil. To guard against trichinosis infection, make sure that pork is thoroughly cooked to a minimum internal temperature of 140° F. Properly cooked pork turns white, with no pink meat.

Like meat, poultry can be cooked using both dry- and moist-heat methods. But if you broil or bake poultry, time it carefully, since the intense heat of broiling or overlong baking will toughen poultry and dry it out. Moist-heat methods yield the most flavorful birds, and long cooking by moist heat will help tenderize older, tougher birds.

The recipes that follow use poultry as well as lean cuts of meat in main dishes, salads, sandwiches and side dishes. While a three-ounce portion of meat or poultry may be less than you are accustomed to eating at a meal, you will feel satisfied because the meat is combined with vegetables and other filling, high-carbohydrate foods.

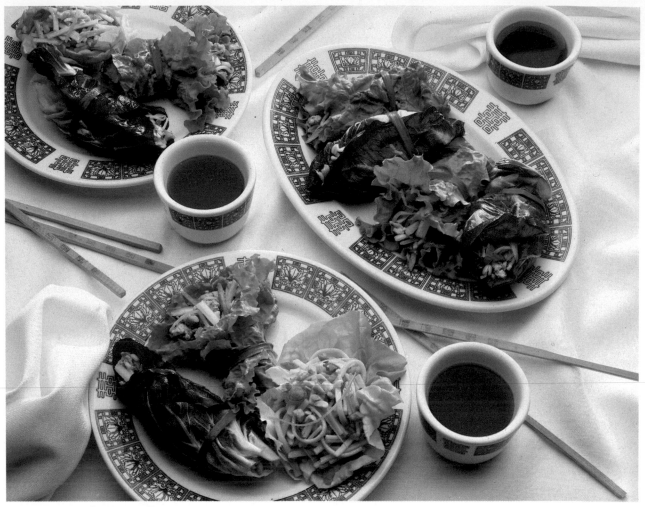

Lettuce-Wrapped Spring Rolls

LETTUCE-WRAPPED SPRING ROLLS

Standard Chinese spring rolls are deep-fried. These, filled mostly with vegetables and wrapped in lettuce, have much less fat and more fiber.

6 ounces linguine-size rice noodles

1 tablespoon plus 1 teaspoon grated fresh ginger

2 tablespoons reduced-sodium soy sauce

2 tablespoons Japanese rice-wine vinegar

1 1/2 tablespoons honey

1 cup shredded carrot

1/2 cup thinly sliced scallions

1 tablespoon cornstarch

1/4 teaspoon salt

2 teaspoons vegetable oil

1/2 pound lean pork loin, finely chopped

2 teaspoons Chinese chili oil

2 garlic cloves

2 cups julienned Napa cabbage

1 cup bean sprouts

12 large lettuce leaves

1 tablespoon chopped unsalted dry-roasted peanuts

CALORIES	368
56% Carbohydrate	52 g
19% Protein	17 g
25% Fat	10 g
CALCIUM	69 mg
IRON	3 mg
SODIUM	500 mg

Bring 2 quarts of water to a boil. Place the noodles in a large heatproof bowl, pour the water over them and set aside 7 minutes. Drain the noodles and cool under cold water. Return 3 cups of noodles to the bowl and add 1 teaspoon of ginger, 1 1/2 tablespoons of soy sauce, 1 tablespoon plus 1 teaspoon of vinegar, 1 teaspoon of honey, 1/4 cup of carrot and 1/4 cup of scallions; toss to combine and set aside. Coarsely chop the remaining noodles; set aside.

In a small bowl mix the cornstarch, salt, the remaining soy sauce, honey, vinegar and 2 tablespoons of water; set aside. Heat the vegetable oil in a wok or large skillet over medium-high heat. Stir fry the pork and remaining scallions 2 minutes, or until the pork is opaque; transfer to a large bowl. Add the chili oil to the wok and stir fry the garlic and remaining ginger 1 minute. Add the cabbage, bean sprouts and remaining carrot, and stir fry 1 minute. Add the cornstarch mixture and cook another minute, then add the vegetable mixture to the bowl with the pork. Stir in the reserved chopped noodles.

Spoon equal amounts of the pork mixture onto each of 8 lettuce leaves and roll the leaves up; divide among 4 plates. Place the remaining leaves on the plates to serve as cups and fill them with the noodle-vegetable mixture. Sprinkle the noodles with chopped peanuts and serve.   Makes 4 servings

STIR-FRIED BEEF WITH VEGETABLES

Unlike most frying methods, stir frying adds little fat to the food: Due to the constant stirring, little oil is needed to keep the food from sticking.

1 cup long-grain white rice	1/4 pound lean beef flank steak, cut
2 tablespoons olive oil	into narrow 3-inch strips
3 tablespoons Japanese rice-wine	6 cups trimmed spinach leaves
vinegar	1/2 cup thinly sliced scallions
5 tablespoons low-sodium beef	3 ounces snow peas, trimmed and
stock	halved diagonally (1 cup)
2 garlic cloves, minced	One 8-ounce can water chestnuts,
1 tablespoon grated fresh ginger	drained
1 tablespoon Chinese five-spice	1 cup thinly sliced radishes
powder	2 cups broccoli florets
1/2 teaspoon salt	

Bring 2 1/2 cups of water to a boil in a medium-size saucepan. Stir in the rice, cover, reduce the heat to low and cook 20 minutes, or until the water is absorbed. While the rice is cooking, in a medium-size bowl combine the oil, vinegar, stock, garlic, ginger, five-spice powder and salt. Add the beef and set aside at room temperature for 30 minutes. Cut the spinach into thin strips by stacking several leaves, rolling them and then cutting them crosswise.

Drain the beef, reserving the marinade. In a wok or large skillet, heat 1 tablespoon of the marinade over high heat. Add the beef and cook 2 minutes; transfer to a small bowl, cover with foil and set aside. Add the remaining marinade to the wok and heat for 30 seconds. Add the scallions, snow peas, water chestnuts, radishes and broccoli, then the spinach, cover and cook 2 minutes, or just until the spinach wilts. Uncover the skillet and stir fry the mixture 2 minutes. Return the beef to the skillet and toss to reheat. Mound the rice on a platter and top with the vegetables and beef.   Makes 4 servings

Note: Chinese (or Oriental) five-spice powder may include anise, star anise, cinnamon, cloves, fennel seeds and/or Szechuan peppercorns. It is sold in the spice section of many supermarkets and in Oriental food stores.

E*ven though some people think that brown eggs are more nutritious than those with white shells, there is no difference between the two (except in the breed of chicken that laid them). Similarly, there are those who claim that fertilized eggs — generally sold in health-food stores — are better for you than the unfertilized variety stocked by supermarkets and groceries. In fact, unfertilized eggs are just as nutritious and generally remain fresh longer. Store eggs in the refrigerator in a covered container to prevent them from picking up odors from other foods.*

CALORIES	328
58% Carbohydrate	48 g
14% Protein	12 g
28% Fat	10 g
CALCIUM	90 mg
IRON	4 mg
SODIUM	352 mg

LIME-MARINATED TURKEY WITH FETTUCCINE

Turkey is a good source of niacin, a B vitamin the muscles need in order to use carbohydrates.

CALORIES	379
67% Carbohydrate	65 g
20% Protein	19 g
13% Fat	6 g
CALCIUM	73 mg
IRON	3 mg
SODIUM	207 mg

1/2 pound boneless turkey breast
Grated peel of 1 lime
3 tablespoons lime juice
1/4 cup low-sodium chicken stock
1 tablespoon rinsed, drained capers
1 cup golden raisins
1/4 teaspoon salt
1/4 teaspoon pepper

1/2 pound fettuccine
1 tablespoon vegetable oil
2 cups julienned cucumber
2 cups green beans, blanched
1 cup julienned carrot, blanched
1 cup sliced white mushrooms
1/4 cup chopped fresh parsley

Bring 1 cup of water to a boil in a medium-size skillet over medium heat. Add the turkey, reduce the heat to low and simmer, uncovered, 15 minutes. Remove the skillet from the heat and let the turkey cool in the cooking liquid. In a large bowl combine the lime peel, juice, stock, capers, raisins, salt and pepper. Drain the turkey, place it in the marinade, cover and set aside to marinate at least 4 hours at room temperature, or overnight in the refrigerator.

Bring a large pot of water to a boil. Cook the fettuccine according to the package directions until al dente; drain, transfer to a large bowl and toss with the oil. Add the vegetables and toss well. Drain the turkey, reserving the marinade, and cut the turkey on the diagonal into thin slices. Divide the fettuccine mixture among 5 plates and arrange the turkey slices on top. Drizzle with the marinade and sprinkle with parsley. *Makes 5 servings*

BEEF, CABBAGE AND BEER SOUP

Fatty cuts of meat are usually more tender than leaner cuts. Here, long cooking and the addition of beer and lemon juice tenderize the lean beef.

1 tablespoon plus 1 teaspoon
    vegetable oil
1/2 pound lean beef, cut into 1-inch
    cubes
6 cups thinly sliced cabbage
1 cup chopped onion
1 teaspoon caraway seeds
1/4 teaspoon black pepper

1 cup tomato purée
1 1/2 cups beer
1/4 cup lemon juice
2 tablespoons honey
3/4 pound potatoes, peeled and
    cut into 1-inch cubes
1/2 teaspoon salt

CALORIES	191
53% Carbohydrate	26 g
23% Protein	11 g
24% Fat	5 g
CALCIUM	59 mg
IRON	2 mg
SODIUM	392 mg

In a large heavy-gauge saucepan or Dutch oven, heat the oil over medium heat. Brown the beef 3 to 5 minutes, or until well browned on all sides. Using a slotted spoon, transfer the beef to a plate and set aside. Add the cabbage, onion, caraway seeds and pepper to the pan. Cook over medium heat, stirring occasionally, about 10 minutes, or until the cabbage is wilted. Stir in 2 cups of water, the tomato purée, beer, lemon juice and honey. Bring the mixture to a boil and return the beef to the pan. Reduce the heat, cover the pan and simmer 30 minutes, stirring occasionally. Add the potatoes, cover and simmer 1 1/4 to 1 1/2 hours, or until the beef is very tender. Just before serving, add the salt, and additional pepper if desired. *Makes 6 servings*

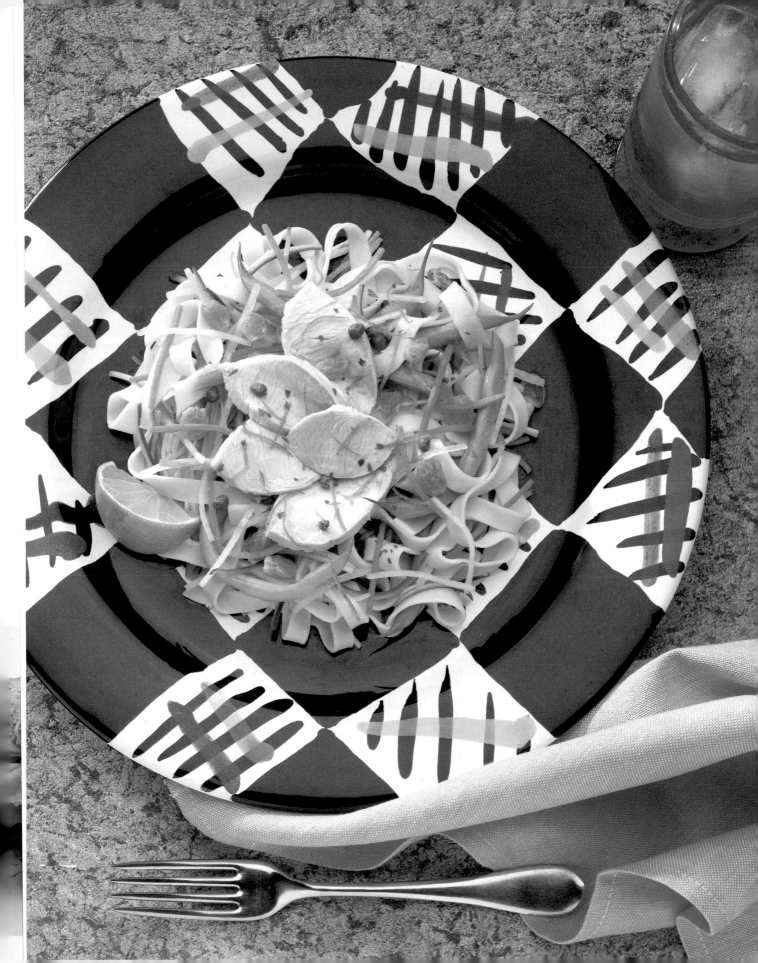

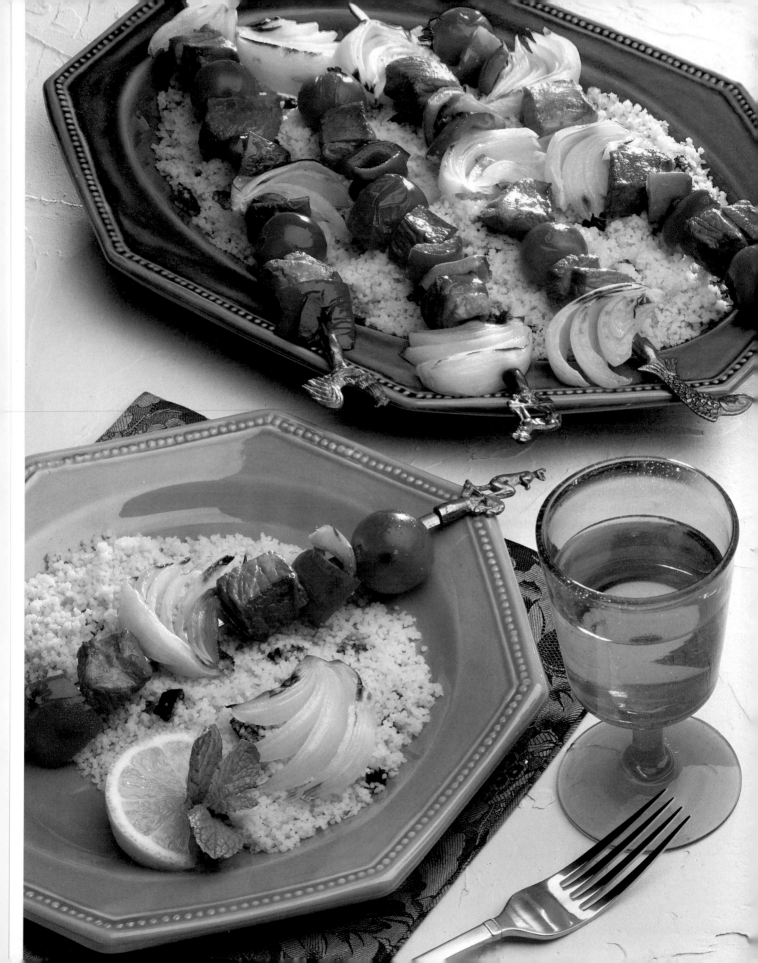

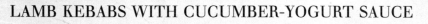

LAMB KEBABS WITH CUCUMBER-YOGURT SAUCE

Three ounces of lamb provides almost 10 percent of the required daily amount of iron in the form of heme iron, which is absorbed more efficiently than the non-heme iron found in vegetables.

3/4 cup lemon juice
2 tablespoons olive oil
2 garlic cloves, minced
1 teaspoon salt
1/2 teaspoon ground cumin
1/4 teaspoon Cayenne pepper
1/2 pound boneless leg of lamb, cut
   into 1-inch cubes
1 medium-size cucumber

1/2 cup plain lowfat yogurt
1/2 cup chopped fresh mint leaves
1 cup couscous
1 pint cherry tomatoes
1 large onion, cut into wedges
1 each green and red bell pepper,
   cut into 1-inch squares
10 prunes, cut into 1/4-inch dice

In a small bowl stir together 1/2 cup of the lemon juice, the oil, garlic, salt, cumin and Cayenne. Add the lamb cubes and set aside to marinate 1 hour at room temperature. Meanwhile, for the sauce, peel, seed, grate and squeeze dry the cucumber; you should have about 1/2 cup. In a small bowl, combine the cucumber, yogurt, mint and remaining lemon juice. Stir well, cover and re-frigerate until ready to serve.

  Fifteen minutes before serving, preheat the broiler. Bring 1 1/2 cups of water to a boil in a small saucepan. Place the couscous in a medium-size heatproof bowl, pour the boiling water over it and cover the bowl tightly; set the couscous aside to steam 10 minutes. Meanwhile, thread the lamb cubes, tomatoes, onion wedges and bell pepper squares alternately on 6 skewers. Broil the kebabs 4 inches from the heat 4 minutes, then turn and broil another 4 minutes. Uncover the couscous and fluff it with a fork. Add the prunes and mix well. Turn the couscous onto a platter, arrange the kebabs on top, and serve the cucumber-yogurt sauce on the side.   Makes 6 servings

CALORIES	289
54% Carbohydrate	37 g
21% Protein	14 g
25% Fat	7 g
CALCIUM	70 mg
IRON	2 mg
SODIUM	418 mg

CALORIES	469
65% Carbohydrate	77 g
18% Protein	22 g
17% Fat	9 g
CALCIUM	69 mg
IRON	4 mg
SODIUM	356 mg

CHINESE CHICKEN SALAD

The white meat from a chicken breast is lower in fat than dark meat. Overall, chicken has substantially less fat than goose or duck.

1/2 pound skinless, boneless chicken breast

2 cups shredded Napa cabbage

1 1/2 cups each julienned red, yellow and green bell pepper

1/4 pound asparagus, blanched and cut into 1-inch pieces

1 cup bean sprouts

1/3 cup lemon juice

1 garlic clove, minced

1 tablespoon finely shredded fresh ginger

1/2 teaspoon red pepper flakes

3 tablespoons reduced-sodium soy sauce

2 tablespoons Oriental sesame oil

1 pound linguine, cooked, drained and cooled

1 small honeydew melon, peeled and cut into thin wedges

Bring 1 cup of water to a boil in a small skillet over medium heat. Add the chicken, reduce the heat to low and simmer 10 minutes. Drain the chicken and set aside to cool.

Cut the cooled chicken into thin strips and transfer it to a medium-size bowl. Add the cabbage, peppers, asparagus and bean sprouts. For the dressing, in a small bowl stir together the lemon juice, garlic, ginger, red pepper flakes, soy sauce and sesame oil. Pour the dressing over the chicken mixture and toss to combine. Mound the linguine on a platter and top with the chicken mixture. Surround the salad with honeydew slices. Makes 6 servings

W*hen you cut raw meat or poultry on a cutting board, you release juices that can serve as a growth medium for harmful bacteria. So after cutting raw meat, wash the board thoroughly with soap and hot water; it should be cleaned periodically with a weak solution of chlorine bleach to kill off any residual bacteria. If possible, keep a separate cutting board for vegetables.*

BEEF ENCHILADAS

The beef in these enchiladas is a good source of phosphorus, the mineral that, along with calcium, is the main component of our bones and teeth.

1 tablespoon olive oil

2 cups finely chopped onion

1 1/3 cups finely chopped green bell pepper

2 cups long-grain white rice

3/4 teaspoon salt

2 teaspoons chili powder

1/2 teaspoon ground cumin

1/4 teaspoon ground coriander

1 cup canned whole tomatoes with their liquid

Eight 6-inch corn tortillas

1/4 teaspoon turmeric

3/4 pound lean beef strip steak

2 cups shredded lettuce

2 medium-size fresh tomatoes, diced

1/2 cup frozen or canned corn kernels

1 medium-size avocado, peeled and thinly sliced

1/2 cup bottled salsa

Heat the oil in a large saucepan over medium-low heat. Add 1 cup of onions and 2/3 cup of peppers and sauté 4 minutes, or until the vegetables are soft. Add the rice, salt and half of the chili powder, cumin and coriander, and cook, stirring constantly, 1 minute. Add 4 cups of water and the canned tomatoes with their liquid, and bring to a boil. Reduce the heat to low and simmer, covered, 20 minutes.

CALORIES	421
58% Carbohydrate	61 g
15% Protein	16 g
27% Fat	13 g
CALCIUM	97 mg
IRON	5 mg
SODIUM	435 mg

Meanwhile, preheat the broiler. Wrap the tortillas tightly in foil and place them on the lower rack of the oven to heat. In a small bowl, combine the turmeric with the remaining chili powder, cumin and coriander. Cut the steak in half lengthwise and sprinkle it on all sides with the chili-powder mixture. Place the steak on a broiler pan and broil it 5 inches from the heat for 3 minutes, then turn the steak and broil it another 2 minutes, or until the juices run pink when the meat is pierced. Turn off the broiler, leaving the tortillas in the oven. Slice the steak into 24 thin strips.

When the rice is cooked, in a large bowl toss together the remaining onions and peppers, the lettuce, fresh tomatoes and corn. Unwrap the tortillas and lay each one on a plate. Spread 1/4 cup of rice on each tortilla and top with 3 strips of steak. Divide the vegetable mixture among the tortillas, garnish with avocado slices and drizzle 1 tablespoon of salsa over each enchilada. Serve the remaining rice on the side. Makes 8 servings

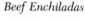

Beef Enchiladas

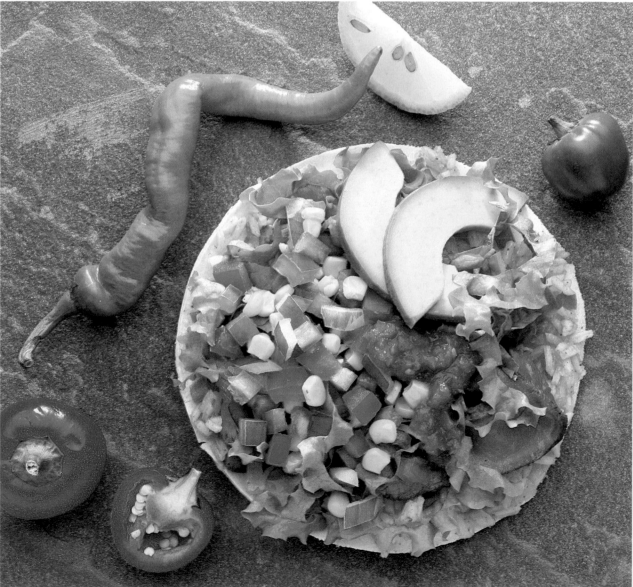

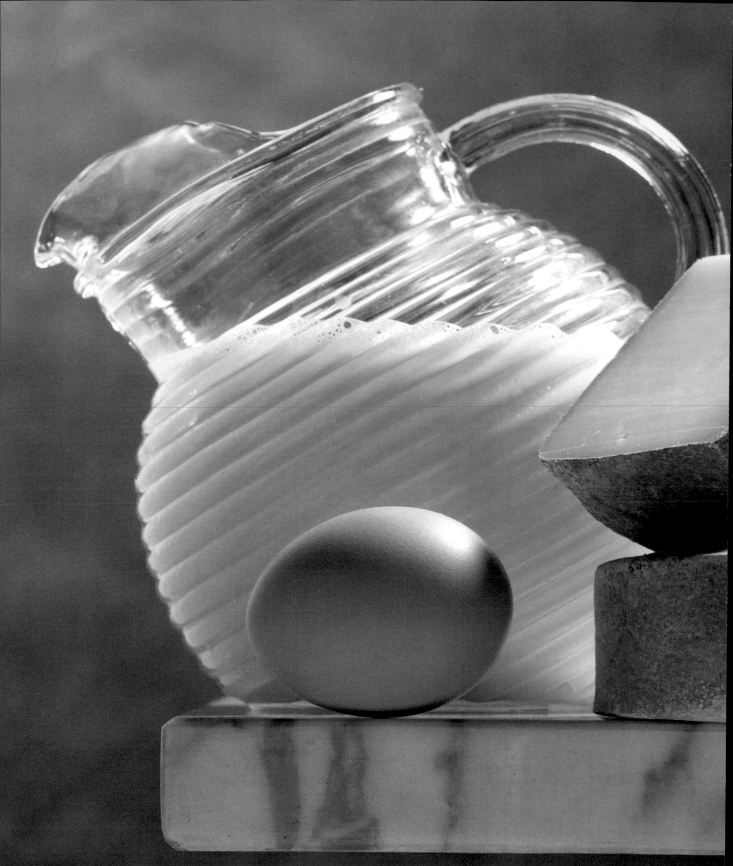

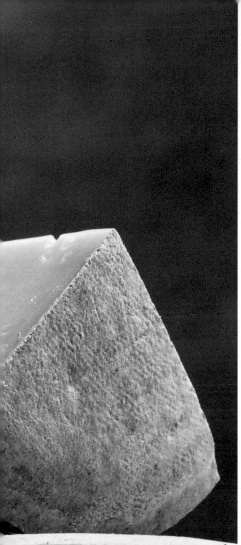

CHAPTER EIGHT

Dairy

An important source of calcium, A, D and B vitamins, and protein for complementing vegetarian dishes

Milk and other dairy products — including buttermilk, cheese and yogurt — are the most important dietary sources of calcium, supplying about three fourths of our intake of this mineral. One cup of milk contains about 300 milligrams of calcium, which constitutes a substantial portion of the 800 milligrams recommended for most adults; and the 1,200 to 1,500 milligrams suggested for pregnant, lactating and post-menopausal women. Although dairy products are the richest source of calcium, other foods can supply significant calcium if eaten in sufficient quantity *(see illustration page 21)*. Calcium is essential primarily for the growth and maintenance of bones and teeth. Yet studies have shown that more than two thirds of American women and up to half of all American men do not consume as much calcium as they should.

Calcium deficiency is an important factor in osteoporosis, a progressive loss of bone density afflicting at least 15 million Americans, mostly older women. Research has shown that consuming adequate calcium — not just in childhood but throughout one's life — may prevent, or at least delay, osteoporosis. Inadequate calcium consumption can also lead to weakening and loss of teeth, and studies have linked low calcium intake to high blood pressure, which affects an estimated 60 million Americans.

Besides supplying calcium, milk and milk products provide most of the other essential nutrients. One cup of milk (whole, lowfat or skim) contains about 15 to 20 percent of the protein an adult needs daily, and it comes in a form that is almost completely absorbed and used by the body. And, because its protein is complete, milk complements legumes, cereals and breads, supplying the two amino acids (lysine and methionine) that these protein sources lack.

The vitamins in whole milk include A and D and the B vitamins. Because skim and lowfat milk lose the fat-soluble vitamins A and D when they are defatted, they are almost always fortified with these substances. Milk contains only a minimal amount of vitamin C, which is further decreased by the high temperatures used in pasteurization. Milk's roster of minerals includes phosphorus, potassium and a very small amount of easily absorbed iron, as well as some magnesium, copper, chlorine and sulfur. Unfortunately, milk also contains a fair amount of sodium, and most cheeses contain a great deal of sodium, which is added during processing.

The most serious drawback to milk is that, in its whole form, it contains a considerable amount of saturated fat. But lowfat milk has about half the fat of whole milk, and skim milk has almost no fat and approximately half the calories of whole milk. Three glasses of skim milk a day provide an adult's daily requirement of 800 milligrams of calcium with just 240 calories, compared to 450 calories for the same amount of whole milk. Skim milk and lowfat milk products such as buttermilk, lowfat yogurt and lowfat cheese (including farmer cheese and skim-milk ricotta) are also preferable to whole-milk products because they have far less fat yet the same nutrients. Most hard cheese is high in fat, so it should be consumed in moderation.

Some people can digest only a small amount of milk because of its lactose (milk sugar) content. This problem occurs because the digestive enzyme lactase, which helps break lactose into its component sugars, is produced in insufficient amounts. Lactose-intolerant individuals suffer from bloating, gas, cramps and diarrhea, the result of the undigested sugar passing through the intestines.

People with lactose intolerance can try consuming more cultured milk products, such as cheese, live-cultured yogurt, buttermilk and acidophilus milk (cultured milk to which special bacteria have been added). In all of these foods, lactose has already been partially broken down by beneficial microorganisms. Even if you consume only cultured milk products, you can still meet your daily calcium requirement. If you have lactose intolerance, avoid eating dairy foods on an empty stomach and limit the amount you consume at one sitting. You can also add packaged lactase to dairy products at home or buy

Buying and Storing Guide

◆ Milk is available in numerous forms. The most common are whole milk (in which fat comprises 48 percent of the calories), lowfat milk (about 30 percent fat calories), skim milk (four percent fat calories), filled milk (milk fat removed and replaced by another type of fat), buttermilk (fermented skim or lowfat milk), yogurt (a fermented product made from either whole or lowfat milk), sour cream (86 percent fat calories), heavy cream (97 percent fat calories), evaporated milk (60 percent of water evaporated, then sealed and sterilized), dry milk (in powder form, all water removed), acidophilus milk (milk whose lactose has been predigested by special bacteria), low-sodium milk (95 percent of sodium removed) and lactase-treated milk (for people with lactose intolerance). Unpasteurized raw milk is sold in some states, but it may contain dangerous bacteria.

◆ Store milk in the container it comes in; keep it in the coldest part of your refrigerator. Exposing milk to light not only changes its flavor, but also destroys its riboflavin. Pasteurized fresh milk will keep up to five days after purchase.

◆ While hard cheese will keep in the refrigerator for several weeks, soft cheese must be used within several days. Wrap hard cheese tightly to protect it from drying out. Hard cheese can be frozen if it is cut into pieces and then tightly wrapped in plastic wrap. Do not freeze soft cheese such as cottage cheese; freezing adversely affects its texture.

milk products that have been treated with lactase. Cultured milk products are not only easier to digest, but they may increase the body's use of calcium. Preliminary evidence also suggests that such products may reduce the risks of large-bowel cancer. Many of the recipes in this volume use lowfat cultured milk products.

Because dairy products are so nutritious, you should incorporate them into as many dishes as possible — at breakfast, lunch and dinner. Take care in cooking them, though: Milk's flavor, odor and texture can be adversely affected by prolonged high-heat cooking. Stir milk often as it cooks, or heat it in a double boiler. And be sure to cover the pan. If you do not, a skin will develop on the surface of the milk, blocking steam release and possibly causing the milk to boil over. If you skim the skin, you will lose valuable nutrients. Milk also tends to scorch and curdle, so cook dishes with milk in them over moderate heat.

You can substitute nonfat dry milk powder for fresh milk in most recipes by sifting it with other dry ingredients and compensating for the loss of liquid with water. Using nonfat milk powder is an easy way to increase the nutritional value of a dish while adding only a few calories to it.

Cheese should be heated over low temperatures to prevent toughening or coagulation. Cheese sauces may separate if overheated. When baking, use moderate oven temperatures and try to add the cheese near the end of the cooking time. Cheese dishes bake better if the baking dish is placed in a pan of hot water, or if the cheese is covered with bread crumbs or another insulating topping.

CALORIES	251
58% Carbohydrate	37 g
14% Protein	9 g
28% Fat	8 g
CALCIUM	144 mg
IRON	1 mg
SODIUM	141 mg

RICOTTA PANCAKES WITH STRAWBERRY SAUCE

The skim-milk ricotta cheese in this breakfast dish has less fat, less cholesterol and fewer calories than ricotta cheese made with whole milk.

1 pint strawberries
2 tablespoons orange juice
1/2 teaspoon grated orange peel
6 tablespoons sugar
2 large eggs, separated
1/2 cup part skim-milk ricotta

1/4 cup lowfat milk (1%)
6 tablespoons unbleached all-purpose flour
1/4 teaspoon baking powder
Pinch of salt
2 teaspoons vegetable oil

For the sauce, wash, dry and hull the strawberries. Place one fourth of the berries in a food processor or blender and process until puréed. Add the orange juice, peel and 4 tablespoons of sugar and process until combined; transfer to a small bowl. Slice the remaining strawberries and stir them into the purée; set aside.

For the pancake batter, combine the egg yolks and ricotta in the food processor or blender and process until smooth. Add the milk, flour, baking powder, salt and the remaining sugar, and process until well blended; transfer to a large bowl. In another large bowl, using an electric mixer, beat the egg whites until they hold stiff peaks but are still moist. Gently fold the egg whites into the batter; set aside.

Heat 1 teaspoon of oil in a large nonstick skillet over medium heat. Using a generous 1/4 cup of batter for each, make 4 pancakes. Cook about 4 minutes, or until the tops are bubbly, then turn them and cook another 3 to 4 minutes, or until the bottoms are golden. Transfer the pancakes to a platter and cover with foil to keep warm. Add the remaining oil to the skillet and make 4 more pancakes in the same fashion. Divide the pancakes among 4 plates and top each serving with some of the strawberry sauce.   Makes 4 servings

VEGETABLE QUESADILLAS

This Tex-Mex version of a grilled cheese sandwich makes a good light lunch or breakfast dish. Quesadillas usually contain quite a bit of high-fat cheese, but here the yogurt provides protein and calcium without much fat.

2 flour tortillas
2 fresh plum tomatoes, sliced
1/2 red bell pepper, finely chopped
1/2 yellow bell pepper, finely chopped
2 scallions, finely chopped

1 large carrot, grated
1/2 cup grated Monterey Jack cheese
1/2 cup plain lowfat yogurt
2 tablespoons bottled salsa
10 watercress sprigs, trimmed

CALORIES	216
43% Carbohydrate	24 g
18% Protein	10 g
39% Fat	10 g
CALCIUM	280 mg
IRON	2 mg
SODIUM	380 mg

Heat a medium-size nonstick skillet over medium heat. Place a tortilla in the skillet and cook 2 to 3 minutes to warm it. Turn it over in the skillet and place half of the tomatoes, bell peppers, scallions and carrot on one half of the tortilla. Top the vegetables with half of the cheese, yogurt, salsa and watercress. Fold the tortilla over the filling and cook another 3 minutes, or until the cheese melts. Transfer the quesadilla to a plate, cover it with foil to keep it warm and make another quesadilla in the same fashion.   Makes 2 servings

Vegetable Quesadillas ▷

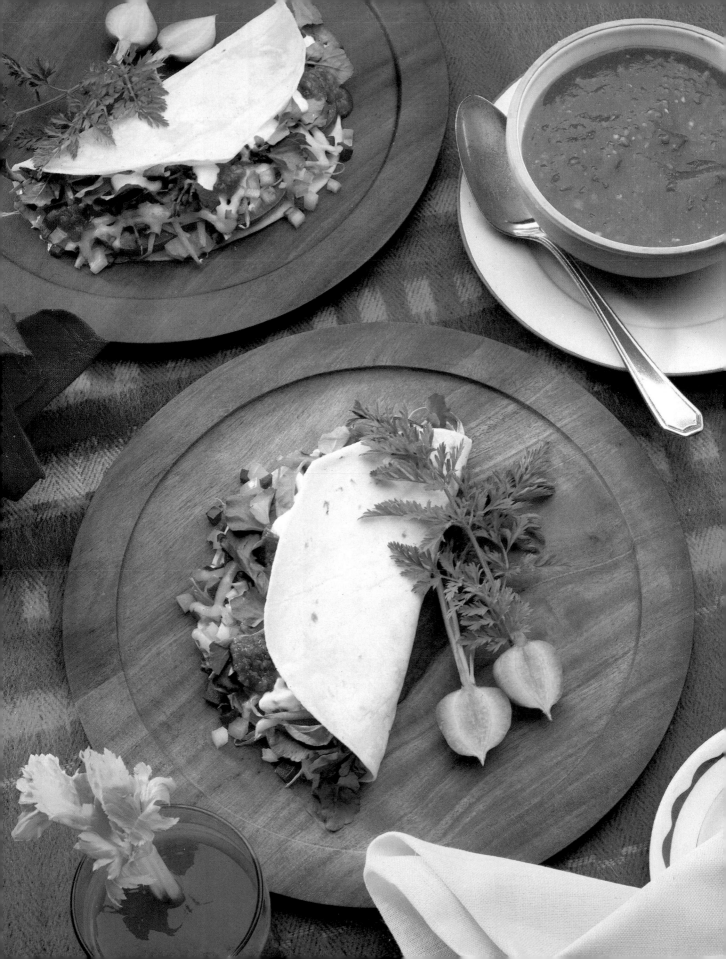

KASHA WITH YOGURT AND BLUEBERRIES

Cooking the kasha in lowfat milk (a complete protein) helps your body make full use of the incomplete protein in the grain.

CALORIES		139
73% Carbohydrate		26 g
20% Protein		7 g
7% Fat		1 g
CALCIUM		226 mg
IRON		1 mg
SODIUM		120 mg

2 cups lowfat milk (1%)
1/2 cup coarse kasha
1/2 teaspoon ground cinnamon
Pinch of salt

1/2 cup plain lowfat yogurt
4 teaspoons brown sugar
1 cup fresh blueberries, or frozen
    blueberries, thawed

In a small saucepan over medium-high heat, bring the milk to a boil. Gradually stir in the kasha, then the cinnamon and salt. Reduce the heat to low and cook, stirring occasionally, about 10 minutes, or until the milk is absorbed. Spoon the kasha into 4 bowls and top each serving with 2 tablespoons of yogurt, a teaspoon of sugar and 1/4 cup of blueberries.   Makes 4 servings

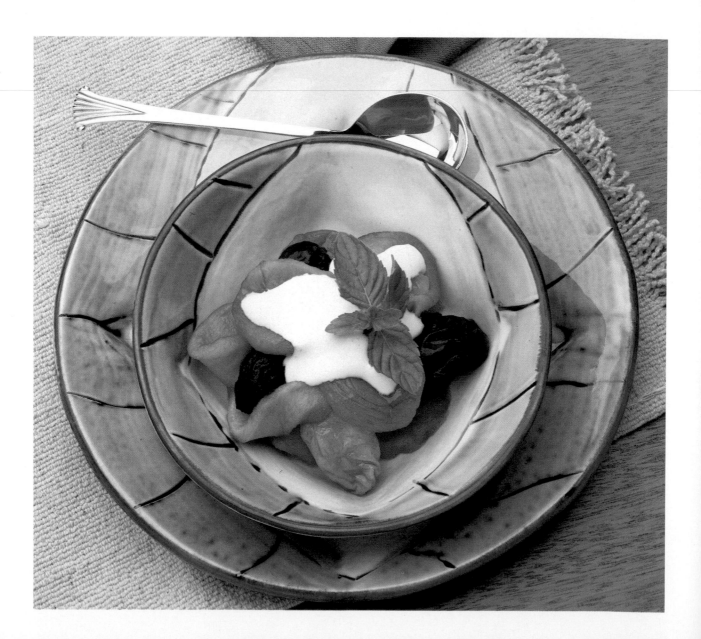

HERBED YOGURT CHEESE WITH POTATO SLICES

Yogurt cheese is an excellent lowfat, low-calorie alternative to cream cheese, which it resembles in texture, appearance and taste. And the warm potato slices are a great improvement, nutritionally speaking, over packaged chips.

CALORIES	101
74% Carbohydrate	19 g
18% Protein	5 g
8% Fat	1 g
CALCIUM	93 mg
IRON	1 mg
SODIUM	34 mg

1 cup plain lowfat yogurt
2 1/2 tablespoons chopped scallion
1 tablespoon chopped fresh dill

1 garlic clove, peeled and pressed
8 small new potatoes (3/4 pound total)

Line a medium-size strainer with dampened cheesecloth and place it over a medium-size bowl. In a small bowl combine the yogurt, scallions, dill and garlic, and stir well. Pour the yogurt mixture into the strainer, cover with plastic wrap and place a small bowl on top. Weight the bowl with a can or other weight. Place the yogurt in the refrigerator overnight to drain.

Twenty minutes before serving, scrub the potatoes and place them in a large pot with cold water to cover. Bring to a boil over high heat, then reduce the heat to low and boil the potatoes 15 to 20 minutes, or until they are easily pierced with a knife. Remove the yogurt cheese from the strainer and mound it in the center of a platter. Cut the potatoes into 1/4-inch-thick slices, arrange the slices around the yogurt cheese and serve immediately.

Makes 4 servings

DRIED FRUIT COMPOTE WITH RICOTTA CREAM

The half cup of part-skim ricotta used in this dessert contains more calcium than a cup of skim milk.

3/4 pound mixed dried fruit
1 cup ruby port
1 cinnamon stick
Four 2 × 1/8-inch strips orange peel
Four 2 × 1/8-inch strips lemon peel

1/4 cup sugar
1/4 cup cream cheese, at room temperature
1/2 cup part skim-milk ricotta cheese
1/4 cup sour cream

In a small nonreactive saucepan combine the dried fruit, port, cinnamon stick, orange and lemon peel and sugar, and bring to a boil over medium-high heat. Reduce the heat to low, cover the pan and simmer 20 minutes. Strain the fruit, reserving the syrup. You should have about 1/4 cup of syrup.

In a medium-size bowl, using an electric mixer, beat the cream cheese until smooth and fluffy. Add the ricotta and beat another 3 minutes. Add the sour cream and reserved port syrup, and beat just until combined. Divide the cooked fruit among 4 bowls and top each serving with 2 tablespoons of the ricotta cream. Serve immediately.

Makes 4 servings

CALORIES	201
70% Carbohydrate	37 g
7% Protein	4 g
23% Fat	5 g
CALCIUM	79 mg
IRON	1 mg
SODIUM	53 mg

◁ *Dried Fruit Compote with Ricotta Cream*

PASTA WITH CREAMY CORIANDER PESTO

The lowfat cottage cheese used in this pasta side dish contains much less saturated fat than the cream and butter often used in pasta sauces. And the cottage cheese contributes a good amount of calcium, too — more than a hard grating cheese such as Parmesan would provide.

2 ounces linguine
1/2 cup lowfat cottage cheese (1%)
1/4 cup fresh coriander leaves
1/2 teaspoon salt
2 1/2 teaspoons olive oil

3 garlic cloves, peeled and thinly sliced
1/4 teaspoon red pepper flakes, or to taste

CALORIES	208
49% Carbohydrate	25 g
22% Protein	11 g
29% Fat	7 g
CALCIUM	62 mg
IRON	1 mg
SODIUM	504 mg

Bring a large pot of water to a boil. Cook the linguine according to the package directions until al dente; drain and set aside. For the sauce, place the cottage cheese, coriander leaves and salt in a food processor or blender and process until smooth; set aside. In a small skillet, heat the oil, garlic and red pepper flakes over very low heat about 5 minutes, or until the garlic is golden. Remove the skillet from the heat, add the linguine and sauce and toss until well combined.

Makes 2 servings

CREAMED ONIONS

Most recipes for creamed onions include a lot of butter as well as whole milk, both of which contain large amounts of saturated fat. This tasty recipe uses lowfat milk and just one teaspoon of butter.

1 pound small white onions, peeled
1 tablespoon sugar
1 teaspoon unsalted butter
1 tablespoon unbleached all-purpose flour

1 cup lowfat milk (1%)
1/8 teaspoon dried sage
1/4 teaspoon salt
2 tablespoons grated Parmesan
1/4 cup chopped fresh parsley

CALORIES	109
62% Carbohydrate	18 g
18% Protein	5 g
20% Fat	2 g
CALCIUM	147 mg
IRON	1 mg
SODIUM	225 mg

In a medium-size skillet, combine the onions, sugar and 3/4 cup of water, and cook over medium heat, tossing occasionally, about 25 minutes, or until most of the liquid has evaporated and the onions are tender and golden. Watch carefully and add a few teaspoons of water if necessary during cooking to prevent the onions from scorching. Remove from the heat and set aside.

Preheat the oven to 375° F. For the sauce, melt the butter in a small saucepan. Whisk in the flour, then gradually whisk in the milk and cook, whisking constantly, about 4 minutes, or until slightly thickened. Rub the sage to a powder between your fingers, then stir it in along with the salt. Transfer the onions to a 1-quart baking dish, pour in the sauce and stir to coat the onions. Sprinkle the onions with Parmesan and bake 10 to 15 minutes, or until the sauce is bubbly and golden. Sprinkle the onions with parsley and serve.

Makes 4 servings

Potato, Cucumber and Bell Pepper Salad with Buttermilk Dressing ▷

POTATO, CUCUMBER AND BELL PEPPER SALAD WITH BUTTERMILK DRESSING

Buttermilk is a lowfat milk product that contains more nutrients (including calcium) than fatty, cholesterol-laden salad binders like mayonnaise.

1 pound new potatoes

1/2 medium-size cucumber

1 red bell pepper

2 garlic cloves, peeled

1 cup buttermilk

2 tablespoons sour cream

2 tablespoons coarsely chopped red onion

1/2 teaspoon salt

1/4 teaspoon pepper

1 tablespoon chopped fresh parsley

Bring a large pot of water to a boil. Scrub the potatoes, cut them into 1-inch cubes and boil them about 15 minutes, or until tender. Meanwhile, peel and seed the cucumber and cut it into large dice. Seed the bell pepper and cut it into 1-inch squares. Bring a medium-size saucepan of water to a boil. Blanch the cucumber 1 minute; remove with a slotted spoon and cool under cold water. Blanch the bell pepper in the same water 2 minutes; remove and cool under cold water. Blanch the garlic 4 minutes; drain and set aside.

Drain the potatoes and set aside to cool slightly. For the dressing, in a food processor or blender combine the garlic with 1/3 cup each of potatoes and buttermilk. Process until puréed, then stir in the sour cream and remaining buttermilk. In a large bowl combine the remaining potatoes, the cucumber, bell pepper and onion. Add the dressing, salt and pepper, and toss gently to combine. Sprinkle the salad with parsley and serve.   Makes 4 servings

CALORIES	141
72% Carbohydrate	26 g
14% Protein	5 g
14% Fat	2 g
CALCIUM	96 mg
IRON	1 mg
SODIUM	350 mg

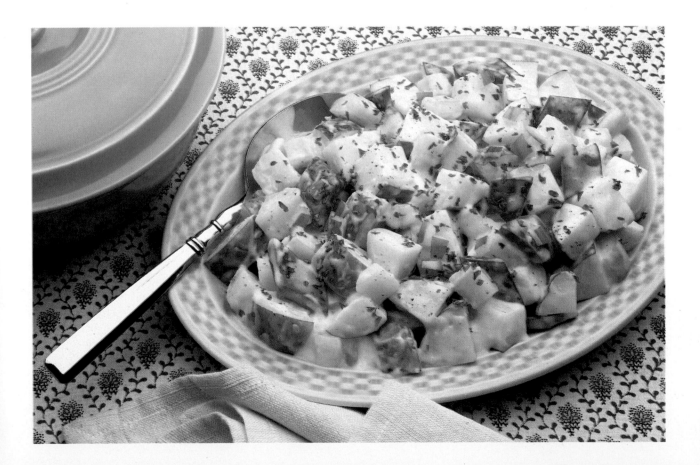

WELSH RAREBIT FONDUE

Skim milk, which is practically fat-free, is the lowest-calorie form of milk available. Cheddar cheese is not a lowfat product, but its robust flavor goes a long way: This fondue has less than one ounce of Cheddar per serving.

CALORIES	242
49% Carbohydrate	29 g
17% Protein	10 g
34% Fat	9 g
CALCIUM	209 mg
IRON	1 mg
SODIUM	382 mg

1/2 cup finely chopped red onion

1 teaspoon olive oil

3/4 cup beer

2 cups shredded sharp Cheddar cheese

1/4 cup fine dry bread crumbs

3 tablespoons unbleached all-purpose flour

1/4 teaspoon Dijon-style mustard

2 teaspoons Worcestershire sauce

1 teaspoon white wine vinegar

3/4 cup skim milk

1/8 teaspoon Cayenne pepper

3/4-pound loaf French bread

2 large apples

In a large skillet over medium-high heat, sauté the onion in the oil about 10 minutes, or until softened. Add the beer, increase the heat to high and cook about 20 minutes, or until the beer has been reduced by half. Pour the contents of the skillet into a food processor and add the cheese, bread crumbs, flour, mustard, Worcestershire sauce, vinegar, milk and Cayenne, and process until smooth. Pour the mixture into a medium-size saucepan and simmer over medium-high heat, stirring often, 8 to 10 minutes, or until the flavors are well blended and the rarebit is hot. Meanwhile, slice the bread and core and slice the apples. Serve the rarebit in a fondue pot or chafing dish, using the bread and apples for dipping.   Makes 10 servings

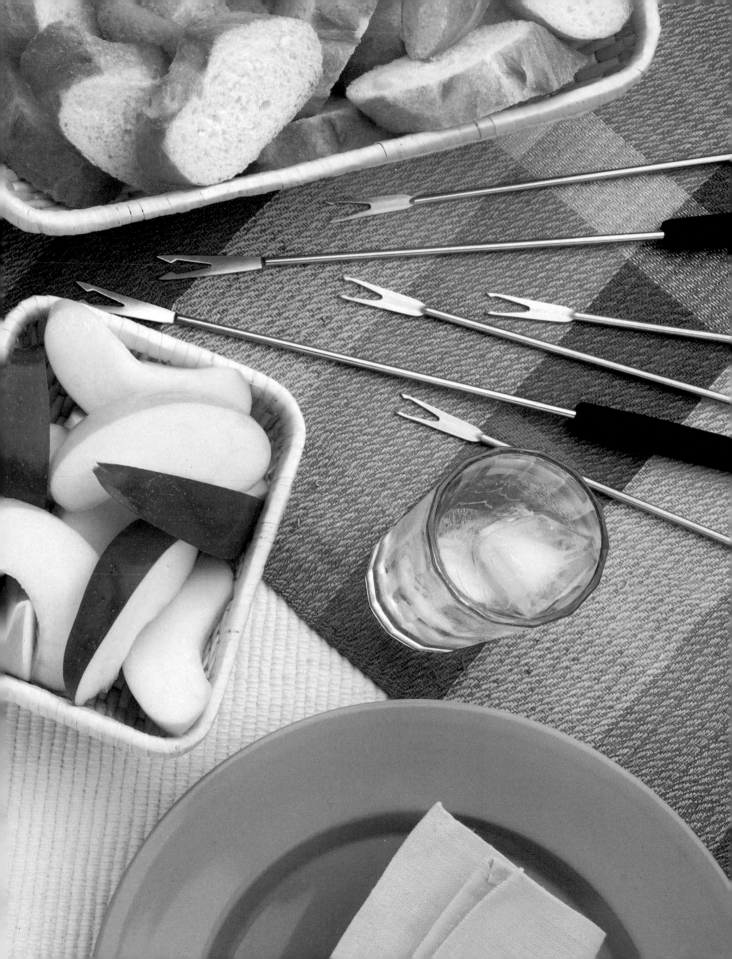

FARMER CHEESE WITH FRUIT ON TOAST

Here is a satisfying alternative to butter or cream cheese on toast. Farmer cheese, which resembles dry-curd cottage cheese, has less than one third the fat of cream cheese and twice the calcium.

CALORIES	229
59% Carbohydrate	37 g
19% Protein	12 g
22% Fat	6 g
CALCIUM	54 mg
IRON	2 mg
SODIUM	355 mg

8 slices whole-wheat bread
3/4 cup farmer cheese
1/4 cup dried apricots, finely
  chopped
2 tablespoons currants

2 tablespoons orange juice
1 tablespoon honey
1/4 teaspoon grated orange peel
1/8 teaspoon vanilla extract

Toast the bread. Meanwhile, preheat the broiler. Place the farmer cheese in a medium-size bowl and mash it with a wooden spoon. Add the remaining ingredients and stir well to blend. Spread the cheese mixture on the toast and broil about 3 minutes, or until the cheese is heated through. Serve immediately.

Makes 4 servings

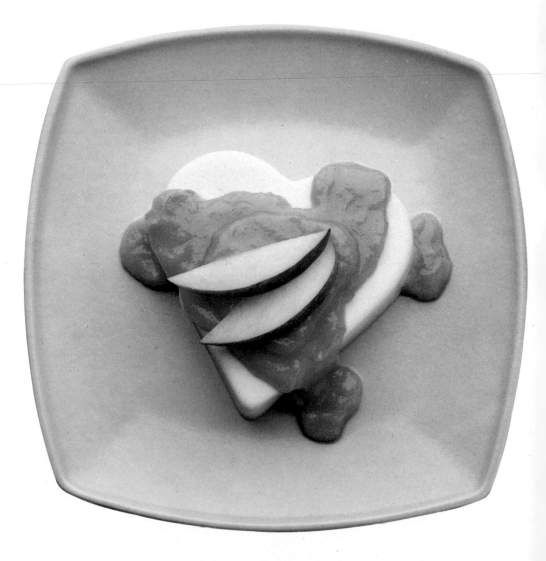

BUTTERMILK-FRUIT DRINK

The fruit in this recipe provides potassium, a mineral that helps maintain the fluid balance in your body. A beverage that replenishes potassium as well as fluids is ideal after strenuous exercise.

1/2 cup dried apricots
1/2 cup drained canned
   juice-packed pears

3/4 cup buttermilk
1/2 medium-size banana
2 ice cubes

CALORIES	343
84% Carbohydrate	78 g
10% Protein	9 g
6% Fat	2 g
CALCIUM	257 mg
IRON	4 mg
SODIUM	205 mg

Quarter the apricots and place them in a small bowl. Add boiling water to cover. Let cool, then refrigerate overnight.

Pour off the excess liquid, then place the apricots in a blender. Process until puréed and return the purée to the bowl. Purée the pears, then add the apricot purée, buttermilk, banana and ice cubes to the blender or processor and process until smooth.

Makes 1 serving

INDIVIDUAL RICOTTA CHEESECAKES
WITH PEACH PUREE

Cheesecake need not include cream cheese, butter or a large quantity of eggs. Lowfat ricotta cheese provides the basis for this rich-tasting dessert.

1 cup dried peaches
1/2 cup plus 1 tablespoon sugar
5 tablespoons plus 1 teaspoon
   lemon juice
1 large egg yolk
1/2 cup skim milk

1 envelope unflavored gelatin
1 teaspoon grated lemon peel
Pinch of salt
1 1/4 cups part skim-milk ricotta
   cheese
1/2 teaspoon vanilla extract

For the peach purée, place the peaches and 3/4 cup of warm water in a medium-size bowl and set aside to soak 30 minutes. Transfer the peaches and soaking liquid to a food processor or blender, add 4 tablespoons of sugar and 4 teaspoons of lemon juice, and purée. Return the purée to the bowl and refrigerate it until well chilled.

Bring enough water to a simmer in the bottom of a double boiler so that the water will not touch the top pan. Combine the egg yolk and milk in the top pan and cook over the simmering water, whisking constantly, about 5 minutes, or until the mixture is light-colored and thick. Stir in the gelatin, lemon peel, salt and remaining sugar, and continue to cook, whisking, about 4 minutes, or until the gelatin dissolves and the custard thickens. Transfer the custard to a large bowl and set aside to cool.

Place the ricotta in a food processor or blender and process until smooth. Add the vanilla and the remaining lemon juice, and process until blended. Gently fold the ricotta mixture into the custard. Spoon the mixture into 4 shallow 4-ounce molds or custard cups. Cover the molds with plastic wrap and refrigerate at least 1 hour. Turn the individual cheesecakes out onto dessert plates and spoon equal amounts of the peach purée over them.

Makes 4 servings

Nondairy creamers usually contain more saturated fat than real cream because they are often made with coconut oil — one of the few vegetable oils that are more saturated than butter, cream or even beef fat. A study of men who were fed diets high in coconut oil showed that the oil raised blood cholesterol. The best choice for lightening your coffee is skim milk.

CALORIES	349
66% Carbohydrate	60 g
15% Protein	14 g
19% Fat	8 g
CALCIUM	268 mg
IRON	2 mg
SODIUM	156 mg

◁ *Individual Ricotta Cheesecakes with Peach Purée*

VANILLA MERINGUE MILK

CALORIES	128
65% Carbohydrate	19 g
33% Protein	10 g
2% Fat	.3 g
CALCIUM	231 mg
IRON	.1 mg
SODIUM	146 mg

This drink is a better lunchtime choice than a milkshake because it is digested more quickly. The high fat content of a milkshake takes a long time to digest, which can slow you down if you exercise after you drink it.

1 1/2 cups skim milk	2 egg whites
2 vanilla beans, split, or 2 teaspoons vanilla extract	4 teaspoons sugar
	Pinch of cinnamon

Combine the milk and vanilla beans in a small saucepan and heat over medium-low heat about 15 minutes. Transfer to a large bowl and set aside 30 minutes, or until completely cooled. Remove and discard the vanilla beans. Refrigerate the milk until well chilled. (If using vanilla extract, simply stir it into cold milk.) Place the bowl of milk in the freezer 1 1/2 to 2 hours, or until the milk thickens and ice crystals just begin to form.

In a large bowl, using an electric mixer, beat the egg whites until foamy. Add the sugar and continue to beat until soft peaks form. Fold half of the egg whites into the milk. Pour the mixture into 2 glasses, top with the remaining egg whites and let stand 10 minutes: The meringue milk will separate into a drinkable consistency. Sprinkle with cinnamon and serve.   Makes 2 servings

Note: Meringue milk can be flavored with almond or rum extract and topped with other spices — nutmeg, for instance — or with finely grated chocolate.

BANANA MOUSSE

CALORIES	249
58% Carbohydrate	36 g
10% Protein	6 g
32% Fat	9 g
CALCIUM	80 mg
IRON	1 mg
SODIUM	48 mg

Calcium and phosphorus, found in dairy foods like yogurt, are the two most important minerals for maintaining strong bones.

4 ripe bananas, peeled	1/2 teaspoon vanilla extract
1 1/4 cups plain whole-milk yogurt	1/2 teaspoon ground ginger
1/4 cup nonbutterfat sour dressing	1/4 cup coarsely chopped toasted almonds
2 tablespoons lemon juice	2 egg whites
6 tablespoons sugar	
1 envelope unflavored gelatin	6 tablespoons unsweetened coconut
3 tablespoons dark rum	

Place the bananas in a food processor or blender and process until puréed: You should have about 1 1/2 cups of purée. Transfer to a medium-size bowl. Add the yogurt, sour dressing, lemon juice and 2 tablespoons of sugar; set aside. Combine the gelatin and rum in a small saucepan and heat over low heat until the gelatin dissolves. Stir the gelatin mixture into the purée, then add the vanilla, ginger and almonds; set aside.

In a large bowl, using an electric mixer, beat the egg whites until soft peaks form. Add the remaining sugar and continue to beat until stiff peaks form. Gently fold the whites into the banana mixture. Pour the mousse into a 5-cup mold or divide it among 6 goblets. Refrigerate the mousse 3 to 4 hours, or until set. Meanwhile, place the coconut in a dry skillet over medium heat and toast it, stirring occasionally, about 2 minutes, or until lightly browned; set aside to cool. Just before serving, sprinkle the mousse with coconut.

Makes 6 servings

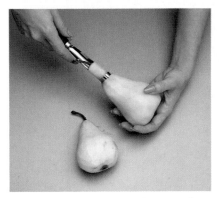

Using an apple corer, core the pears down to but not through the bottom to form a hollow for the cheese filling.

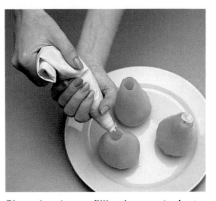

Place the cheese filling in a pastry bag fitted with a plain tip, then pipe the cheese into the hollows in the pears.

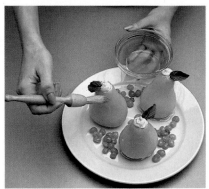

Using a pastry brush, brush the pears with the heated syrup, then garnish the stem end of each pear with a mint leaf.

POACHED PEARS WITH BLUE-CHEESE FILLING

Many of the vitamins in fruit are protected by the skin, so do not peel the pears until you are about to cook them.

3 firm, ripe Bosc pears
1 1/2 cups dry white wine
1/3 cup sugar
2 tablespoons golden raisins

3 ounces Roquefort or other blue
  cheese
4 fresh mint leaves for garnish

Peel the pears and, using an apple corer, core them through the stem end to form a hollow for the filling *(above)*. Place the pears, wine and sugar in a medium-size nonreactive saucepan, cover and poach over medium-low heat, turning the pears occasionally, 25 minutes. Add the raisins and continue cooking another 20 minutes, or until the pears are just tender. (The cooking time will vary with the ripeness of the pears.) Reserving the poaching liquid, remove the pears from the pan and set them aside to cool.

Place the cheese in a small bowl and, using a wooden spoon, cream it until soft and fluffy. Transfer the cheese to a pastry bag fitted with a large plain tip and pipe it into the hollows in the pears *(above)*. Stand the pears on a platter. Return the poaching liquid to medium-high heat and cook, uncovered, about 10 minutes, or until it becomes syrupy. Brush the pears with the syrup, garnish each pear with a mint leaf and spoon the raisins around the platter. Serve some syrup and raisins with each pear.   Makes 3 servings

CALORIES	305
67% Carbohydrate	53 g
9% Protein	7 g
24% Fat	9 g
CALCIUM	179 mg
IRON	1 mg
SODIUM	402 mg

PROP CREDITS

Pages 34-35: plate–Gear, New York City, fork–Gorham, Providence, R.I., bowl–The Hall China Co., New Rochelle, N.Y.; page 41: plates–Ad Hoc Housewares, New York City, linens–Ad Hoc Softwares, New York City; page 42: plate–Gear, New York City, linens–Broadway Panhandler, New York City; page 48: plate–Mood Indigo, New York City, linens–Ad Hoc Softwares, New York City, glass–courtesy of Michael Aron; pages 50-51: plates, bowls–Buffalo China, Inc., Buffalo, N.Y., flatware, napkin holder–Mood Indigo, New York City, salt and pepper shakers courtesy of Bonnie Slotnick, tile–Nemo Tile, New York City, linens–The Pottery Barn, New York City; page 54: knife–J.A. Henckels Zwillingswerk, Inc., Elmsford, N.Y., bowl–The Hall China Co., New Rochelle, N.Y.; page 59: plate–Gear, New York City; page 61: bowl courtesy of Steven Mays; page 65: bowl, spoon–The Pottery Barn, New York City; pages 68-69: plate–Frank McIntosh at Henri Bendel, New York City, flatware–Gorham Sterling, Providence, R.I.; page 71: platter–Gear, New York City, plates–Kuttner Antiques, New York City, linens–Ad Hoc Softwares, New York City; page 74: glasses, swizzle stick–Topeo, New York City; page 81: soup tureen, plates–Deruta of Italy Corp., New York City; page 84: platter, flatware, salt shaker courtesy of Bonnie Slotnick, linens–Ad Hoc Softwares, New York City; page 87: serving bowl, plates–Amigo Country, New York City, glass–Gear, New York City; pages 88-89: platter, plates, flatware, salt and pepper shakers–Mood Indigo, New York City; pages 102-103: plates–Pierre Deux, New York City, glasses–Amigo Country, New York City; page 105: plate–Amigo Country, New York City; page 107: plates–Ad Hoc Housewares, New York City, flatware–Gorham Sterling, Providence R.I., glass–Platypus, New York City, linens–Ad Hoc Softwares, New York City; pages 108-109: tile–Nemo Tile, New York City; page 112: platter, plates, teacups–Buffalo China, Inc., Buffalo, N.Y.; page 115: plate, napkin–Creative Resources, New York City; pages 120-121: platter, plates–Pierre Deux, New York City, linens–Ad Hoc Softwares, New York City; page 124: pitcher–Mood Indigo, New York City; page 129: blanket–Ad Hoc Softwares, New York City; page 130: plate, bowl–Patrick Loughran, New York City, spoon–Gorham Sterling, Providence, R.I.; page 133: tablecloth–Pierre Deux, New York City; pages 134-135: plate, linens–The Pottery Barn, New York City; page 136: plate–Dan Levy, New York City.

ACKNOWLEDGMENTS

Washing machine and dryer supplied by White-Westinghouse, Columbus, Ohio

Index prepared by Ian Tucker

Production by Giga Communications

PHOTOGRAPHY CREDITS

All photographs by Steven Mays, Rebus, Inc.

ILLUSTRATION CREDITS

Page 8, illustration: designed by Brian Sisco, illustrated by David Flaherty; page 11, illustration: designed by Brian Sisco, illustrated by David Flaherty; page 12, chart: Brian Sisco; page 13, illustration: David Flaherty; page 14, illustration: designed by Brian Sisco, illustrated by David Flaherty; page 18, illustration: Brian Sisco; page 21, illustration: David Flaherty; page 23, illustration: Brian Sisco; page 24, chart: Brian Sisco.

Time-Life Books Inc. offers a wide range of fine recordings, including a Rock 'N' Roll era series. For subscription information, call 1-800-445-TIME, or write TIME-LIFE MUSIC, Time & Life Building, Chicago, Illinois 60611.

RECIPE INDEX

Use the following index to help you plan your meals ahead of time. Many of the dishes in the lunch category would also make good light dinners, and soups and salads can often be meals in themselves.

INDEX